Sex and Cancer

Sex and Cancer

Intimacy, Romance, and Love after Diagnosis and Treatment

Saketh R. Guntupalli
Maryann Karinch

ROWMAN & LITTLEFIELD
Lanham · Boulder · New York · London

Published by Rowman & Littlefield
A wholly owned subsidary of The Rowman & Littlefield Publishing Group, Inc.
4501 Forbes Boulevard, Suite 200, Lanham, Maryland 20706
www.rowman.com

Unit A, Whitacre Mews, 26-34 Stannary Street, London SE11 4AB

British Library Cataloguing in Publication Information Available

Library of Congress Cataloging-in-Publication Data

Names: Guntupalli, Saketh R., 1978– author. | Karinch, Maryann, author.
Title: Sex and cancer : intimacy, romance, and love after diagnosis and treatment /
Saketh R. Guntupalli and Maryann Karinch.
Description: Lanham : Rowman & Littlefield, [2017] | Includes bibliographical
references and index.
Identifiers: LCCN 2017002442 (print) | LCCN 2017009526 (ebook) | ISBN
9781442275089 (cloth : alk. paper) | ISBN 9781442275096 (electronic)
Subjects: LCSH: Cancer—Patients—Sexual behavior. | Women—Diseases—
Psychological aspects. | Cance—Complications.
Classification: LCC RC262 .G86 2017 (print) | LCC RC262 (ebook) | DDC
616.99/4—dc23
LC record available at https://lccn.loc.gov/2017002442

♾️™ The paper used in this publication meets the minimum requirements of American
National Standard for Information Sciences—Permanence of Paper for Printed Library
Materials, ANSI/NISO Z39.48-1992.

Printed in the United States of America

To all women who have faced cancer and risen above it

Contents

Disclaimer

The stories presented in this book are based on true events. However, except as specified, names and specific details have been changed at the request of interviewees who wish to remain anonymous. Therefore, any likeness that might be found with any living individual, except as specified, is unintended.

This book is not intended as a substitute for the medical advice of physicians. The reader should regularly consult a physician in matters relating to his or her health and particularly with respect to any symptoms that may require diagnosis or medical attention.

Foreword:
We Are a Team

Camille Grammer

The Foundation for Women's Cancer (FWC) awarded *Real Housewives of Beverly Hills* star Camille Grammer with the 2016 Public Service Award at the 7th National Race to End Women's Cancer on November 6, 2016.

Cancer runs in my family, but so does the strength to fight it. This book captures that kind of fighting spirit and the victories that women create to live renewed lives as beautiful, loving, and fully sexual beings.

My grandmother, mother, and I share many things, but one that we didn't want to share was a genetic predisposition to certain types of cancer. My grandmother battled endometrial cancer while my mother faced the devastating diagnosis of stage III ovarian cancer when she was just forty-seven. Then when I was forty-four, my doctor told me the horrible news: "Camille, you have stage II endometrial cancer."

The first thing that happens is shock. Shortly after that, it's a radical hysterectomy. For someone of my age, that meant instant menopause. Then while the scars are still fresh, the chemotherapy starts. And just to make sure the evil cells are killed, there's internal radiation.

What's after that? Maybe a short pity party, and then we do what most women do: try to be there for our family, tell our friends what the symptoms are, and be grateful the ordeal is over.

But it's vitally important that we do one more thing: take care of ourselves so we return to full womanhood.

Below-the-belt cancers, as I often call them, not only threaten women's lives, but they also force women to go through a harsh transition—first losing a sense of femininity, and then struggling to regain it. In the meantime, at a time when we most need the reassurance of an intimate relationship, we don't have the self-esteem or energy to enjoy one.

This book is all about improving the experience of that transition. It's about revitalizing intimacy, love, and romance after a cancer diagnosis and treatment.

I started taking dance classes to feel feminine. I put on a bikini and decided to feel proud of my body—scars and all. I'm not just a survivor in my body and soul, I'm a thriver, and so are you if you are reading this book.

I am part of your team, cheering you on as you heal and regain your sense of total womanhood. So are all of the women who contributed to this book and all of the partners and children who are thrilled to have you alive. So are all of the women and men who support and participate in the events of the Foundation for Women's Cancer.

We are a team!

Acknowledgments

$\mathscr{T}$his work is the culmination of the many stories, bravery, and courage of women with gynecologic cancer, a group of diseases that affects the very heart of womanhood. These diseases collectively affect over one hundred thousand women a year in the United States and continue to be a source of despair, worry, and concern to women around the world. Our goal continues to be to find cures for these dreadful diseases so our mothers, daughters, wives, and sisters can live burden-free from these devastating illnesses.

No book is written in isolation and without the tireless efforts of the many physicians and staff who take care of women with cancer. This work would not be possible without them. To the staff of nurses, therapists, nutritionists, and medical assistants at the University of Colorado, I offer my most heartfelt thanks and appreciation. I particularly want to thank my research associates Dina Flink, PhD, and our statistician, Jeanelle Sheeder, for their tireless dedication to making this work come to fruition. My coinvestigators at the other institutions that provided the patient data and stories are also held in my highest esteem for their passion and dedication to women's health. Thank you also to the Patty Brisben Foundation for your support of our research.

—Saketh Guntupalli, MD

Thank you to Jim McCormick, first and foremost, for being my primary source of support in every way throughout this project. I also want to say what a great pleasure it is to work in partnership with someone as gifted, sincere, and passionate about his life's work as Saketh Guntupalli, my healer and my friend. We greatly appreciate the contributions of patients and friends who contributed the stories that bring the information in this book to life; you know who you are, and we send you hugs along with our thanks. We also could not have done this without the expert contributions from Dr. Julia Bunning, Dr. Lisa Ruppert, Dr. Jenni Skyler, Trevor Crow Mullineaux, Amber Knuthson, Lisa Falsetto, and Jeanene Smith. Your kindness in sharing your knowledge and your time with us will help improve the lives of our readers. Thank you to our editor, Suzanne Staszak-Silva, and the entire team at Rowman & Littlefield; we appreciate your belief in us and support of our efforts throughout the process. We also want to acknowledge the contributions to our understanding of people we have not yet met but whose knowledge and wisdom we deeply appreciate, especially Brené Brown, the vulnerability guru; author/activist Eve Ensler; psychotherapist/author Esther Perel; and neuroscientist and stress expert Robert Sapolsky. I also want to thank my dear, dear friends and family members who were always there for me in the early days of this process; you know who you are, and you know what I mean! A special thanks also to my wonderful, enthusiastic PEO Sisters in Chapter IY—you're a blessing.

—Maryann Karinch

Introduction:
What Hope Does This Book Give You?

The impetus for this book is a study on sexual function that originated with the Department of Obstetrics and Gynecology at the University of Colorado.

When we saw the study results, we knew we needed to do two things. First, we felt compelled to tell women who had experienced breast or gynecologic cancers that they had *a lot* of company if they had big disruptions in their intimate relationships after diagnosis and treatment. Second, we needed to tell them how to establish a "new normal" in sexual functioning—one that could be even better than before cancer entered their life. With that latter goal in mind, we interviewed therapists who work with women, and in some cases couples, who have struggled with sexual functioning or just wanted to kick their love life into a higher gear. We also talked with many female cancer patients and, whenever possible, their partners or spouses.

If you are reading this book, it's highly likely that you are part of a couple that has gone through cancer. You may love each other as much, or more, than you did prior to being forced to reckon with cancer. But as we found out, loving does not imply normal sexual functioning.

In the interest of full disclosure, we the authors knew each other well before starting work on this book. Saketh is Maryann's gynecologic oncologist. We wanted to make that clear so that you know this isn't "just" a physician and an author teaming up to write a book. This is the deeply personal mission of a team with day-to-day experience—from the perspective of oncologist and patient—of sexual dysfunction after cancer diagnosis and treatment.

The book is divided into two parts, with the first being focused on understanding why cancer and its treatments are bound to affect sexual functioning. There's no way around the challenges, but understanding the various causes of them will go a long way to helping you use the menu of solutions, which are the focus in the second part of the book.

We begin sequentially by exploring the physical changes induced by the disease and treatments for it. Here's something very positive to consider: the treatments keep getting better. For example, a new class of drugs that essentially helps DNA repair itself has proven effective with a number of ovarian cancer patients, particularly those with the BRCA gene (BReast CAncer susceptibility gene) mutation. Another bit of good news is that there are many helpful products on the market to mitigate the side effects of treatments; one of the new ones is a cold cap, which can prevent hair loss during chemotherapy. Many women would give that one a standing ovation!

The answer to "What happens next?" necessitates delving into the mechanics of sex. We realized that, if we going to talk about sexual dysfunction—whether it's caused by physical or psychological reasons—it's important to have a baseline for that discussion. We also introduce a critical concept in this chapter; that is, that sexual intimacy should not be defined only as intercourse. Dr. Jenni Skyler, a sex therapist and founder of the Intimacy Institute, originated one of the most delightful, and useful, metaphors we came across that relates to this concept. Skyler introduces her clients to the Cheesecake of Pleasure, with each slice being a different kind of sexual experience; we delve into this more toward the end of the book.

Our chapter on "issues and answers" centers on the study conducted by the University of Colorado and carried out at four locations, including two UC facilities, Columbia University Medical Center in New York and Loma Linda University Medical Center, which is about sixty miles east of Los Angeles. We reference other studies as well to give you a sense of what kinds of test instruments have been used to ascertain the extent to which sexual function or dysfunction occurs in populations affected by cancers of different kinds. At first glance, that probably sounds dry, but there is a lot of provocative information there. These studies have helped us get a firm grasp of the nature of the dysfunctions and how to address them. They also illuminate how the medical community might avert problems for new patient populations.

Next, we plunge into a discussion of stress. If you want to point a finger at one outcome of a cancer diagnosis and treatment that causes long-lasting, devastating effects on sexual function, it would be stress. Renowned stress expert Robert Sapolsky of Stanford University has demonstrated four major ways that rats deal with stress—and they tell us a lot about how cancer patients might sometimes see themselves as "rats in a lab."

The wrap-up for Part I is the story of Allis and Craig. What they experienced is the most compelling story we encountered in our numerous interviews. How they overcame colossal challenges to create a "new normal" is the most inspiring story we encountered. Allis and Craig point the way toward sexual intimacy despite the odds and help us cross the bridge into the prescriptive part of the book.

Part II is solutions—lots and lots of solutions. Contributors to this section are both patients and experts, with the experts including specialists in pelvic floor rehabilitation, sex therapy, couples counseling, and much more. We get specific about both the psychological/emotional and the physical ways to address myriad problems standing between you and a fulfilling sex life. We also find ways to remind you of the message of one breast cancer survivor's husband: "All people have a lot of things in their life that they did—and they can't believe they did them. Hooray for all of us."

Part II could help any couple overcome intimacy challenges. But our focus is you—women and couples who are going through, or have gone through, the cancer experience and want a thriving, full-bodied love life.

As you begin the book, keep two thoughts in mind:

1. Our immune systems are designed to thrive with connection—intimate connection. The hormones that feed our well-being can be released with a hug from a loved one. Sexual intimacy boosts that production of healthful hormones.
2. Humans are unique among animals because both genders can enjoy sex any time of the month. Three of the most sensitive parts of a woman's body are her lips, nipples, and clitoris, with the clitoris containing an amazing eight thousand nerve endings. There is an obvious practical reason why a human being's hands are sensitive, but the only reason these other three areas are so receptive to sensation is pleasure.

We are designed for pleasure.

I

UNDERSTANDING THE IMPACT

· 1 ·

What Happens First?

*F*irst, you change—physically, biochemically, and psychologically. You change because of the cancer as well as the treatments for it.

Stories from real women and their partners document the changes from just before the diagnosis through all the other stages of their experience. These stories bring the information in this book to life. They convey the secrets, emotions, and practical advice of women who have had a cancer diagnosis, and then went on to discover what that meant for their love life.

There is a large body of data that shows that patients who are in intimate, strong relationships have better survival than patients that are not. This fact is why we sought to collect stories from women who had enlightening insights about both sexual dysfunction after cancer as well as renewed sexual intimacy.

Here's the really good news: The women who contributed their stories—and some of these stories will suck the air out of you and make your heart race—survived. Conquered. Hoped.

The opening story has great personal significance for us because it embodies the compelling reason why we wanted to reach out to all women who have experienced cancer and say, "The 'emperor of all maladies' does not rule your love life." For that reason, we wanted the story to be in the first-person voice of the patient's oncologist:

When Shannon came into my office five years ago, I didn't realize the impact that she would have on my practice, my career, or on my life. The innocuous encounter, something that I have done hundreds of times in my career, seemed quite perfunctory: a second-opinion consult on a patient with ovarian cancer.

As Shannon began the long story—the story that so many cancer survivors have—I began to realize that this interaction was different. Shannon related her story, which began with a small pain in her side that started out innocuously but grew to be a persistent burn. Like most mothers of two, she regarded the pain as more of a pesky annoyance than a life-threatening issue. The pain grew, but through baseball games, homework, and twilight matinee movies she continued, like most mothers, to bear the pain and ignore her health.

Her husband, Paul, seemed unimpressed. He dismissed her vented aches as weakness and gave her the proverbial, androgen-laced "tough it out, honey." While dressing for her husband's annual Christmas party, she noticed that her dress fit tighter, even though she had lost two pounds the previous month. Her husband, oblivious to the nuances of her body after thirteen years of marriage, hardly noticed, and simply asked her to hurry up before they were late. During the drive, Shannon clutched her side like a designer purse as the pain began to increase, but as a good and dutiful wife, she made no reference to it. Evenings like this with her husband were a rare commodity, and she was not going to let a stomach ache get in the way of that.

After they returned home, children asleep in bed and baby sitter dismissed, she cuddled with her husband. The pinot grigio for her and the martini for him had created just the right mood. Their lovemaking was perfunctory, but still pleasant although the nagging pain in her side brought her reality into focus.

Weeks passed in a similar manner. The pain waxed and waned like the moon. Some days it was intense, causing her to stop her chores, and on others, it faded to a dull annoyance. She discussed the pain with a nurse friend of hers who told her to keep exercising and eat right—a dismissive undercurrent of a conversation that hurt her feelings, though she would never tell her.

After about two months and becoming increasingly nauseated, Shannon finally made the journey to her general practitioner's office. Dr. Wheeler had been her trusted confidant for years, knowing things about her even her husband failed to know, like an unplanned pregnancy at age seventeen, treatment for chlamydia two years later, and the small mass in her breast last year that ended up being nothing. She related her symptoms: a vague abdominal pain, mild nausea, and feeling like her clothes were tighter.

This was not Dr. Wheeler's best day. Shannon saw the list of forty patients on the wall and knew there would be a wait. However, his response of "It's just colitis" was surprising. She got a prescription for a laxative and was sent on her way. The usual hug at the end of encounter was discontinued in place of the next patient in the next room.

Two months passed and now Shannon's pain decided to take a journey to the other side of her belly. Except now the pain was a constant reminder that something was wrong. The desire for morning pastries and coffee that had punctuated her morning routine was gone, replaced by an aversion for food that she had not known since she was a child. Shannon knew—she just knew—there was something wrong with her body. She could time her activities of daily living like clockwork, and that clock was grossly undertimed. Nothing seemed to work. She would not have a bowel movement for days, and then diarrhea for a week. An unladylike belch now came so frequently that she was giving her nine-year-old son a run for his money. An appointment in Dr. Wheeler's office was three weeks away, and each passing day seemed an eternity of pain, nausea, and malaise. Even her husband—normally her rock of stoicism—was growing worried.

Shannon made the journey to the emergency room—of course *after* she dropped her children off at school and after her husband went to work—to get things figured out. She related the symptoms to the on-call doctor, a woman who was her age and seemed to grasp the importance of these issues. Yet again, she heard the preliminary diagnosis of colitis. Except this time Shannon was insistent: "Doctor, something isn't right. I don't feel well."

Moved by Shannon's insistence, the doctor relented and ordered a CT scan, a reflex action by most ER doctors that's done not so much for investigative intent but rather to disquiet an insistent patient. As Shannon was wheeled to the machine, she felt the apprehension of all patients who know—with every fiber in their body—that their life would change once they came out off the scanner. She thought about how this would affect her children most of all. Would she be there for them to watch the milestones that make every parent proud? Would she be able to take photos of graduations, first jobs, first cars, girlfriends, and weddings? The forty-minute wait was agony, yet a sense of relief seemed palpable. Perhaps finally a diagnosis.

As the young doctor entered the room, Shannon didn't need to hear anything. The litany of horrors began. There were two masses in her ovaries as well as a mass in something called the omentum [a fatty layer in the pelvic area]—Shannon scanned her memory banks from high school biology, never recalling such a structure—as well as fluid around her stomach. The doctor said that they were suspicious about ovarian cancer but could not be sure. While the apprehension had prepared Shannon to some extent for the diagnosis, it still hit her like a tire iron to the head. And then her brain tortured her on the long drive home. How did this happen to me? Why me? I'm a good person! Why do I deserve this? I'm healthy—this can't be right? What will happen to my children?

When she arrived home, Shannon was emotionally spent. An hour of crying had numbed her temporarily to both the physical and emotional pain. Surprisingly, her husband was home early from work. Glued to the television set, she had sunk into the sofa. He didn't really notice the baggy eyes, smeared makeup, or whimpering for a few minutes. When Shannon felt she had waited long enough, she switched off the TV and told her husband what happened. She expected the perfunctory hug and kiss, the reassurances and the obligatory "We will fight this." Yet a strange and odd thing happened. Paul, who had always been a source of strength, seemed unfazed, almost uncaring. He had the standard questions "Are they sure? Are you going to be okay? Did you like your doctor?" But an emotional response—what Shannon craved the most—seemed lacking.

Paul left the room and got in his car. Shannon initially thought of this as a classic male response. Paul was the stereotypical male in every sense of the word and rarely talked about his feelings. Strangely, this is what had drawn Shannon to him initially. He projected a masculine strength and sense of authority that she had craved. It often meant he stayed an arm's length away from emotional intimacy, but she had accepted him for this flaw. Yet now, at the point she was at the most vulnerable, she needed—no, required—a gentle strength. She craved his arms around her in a way that only her cherished partner would understand. After Paul came back four hours later, he apologized. He said he needed some time to digest and said they would get through it. She finally had the reassurances she needed.

That night, in her desperation to feel some bit of normalcy, she embraced her husband. He turned over to his side, turning his back to her. She was reminded of a time she was forced to share a bed with her brother at a wedding a few years ago; the interaction was all about avoidance, not connection. This would persist for the following weeks.

When she met her surgeon, she learned she would require a "debulking surgery." It made her feel like a cardboard box being shipped around. She would also have to undergo weeks of chemotherapy.

After surgery, she had a traumatic six-day hospital stay in which she had more tubes in her than the infamous Borg characters from *Star Trek*.

Paul grew more and more distant. The kisses that came so naturally to him when he came home from work were gone. Their lovemaking had ceased to exist with minimal embraces or kisses at night. Paul showed up every day after surgery and for each chemotherapy, stood right by her side and dutifully picked up her antinausea medications. After three months, Shannon began to feel right again. She made overtures and dropped subtle (and not-so-subtle hints) about her need to be with Paul intimately. She craved him in a way she hadn't since they dated thirteen years previously. She suspected infidelity but found no substantive clues; his schedule remained unchanged. When she brought the subject of sex up with him, he told her he just needed time and she should focus on healing.

Six months after completing chemo, Paul and Shannon went to their oncologist's office for her checkup. She had been told that if she could get through the first few months without a recurrence her chances were good for a durable remission. She still wasn't quite 100 percent after being loaded up with chemotherapy for sixteen weeks, but she was running again, back to her normal weight, and encouraged by the return of her stamina. The first visit after six months was one of the most apprehensive she had had; she came in worrying she might get the worst possible news—that the battle was still on.

For Shannon, the news was all good; her imaging showed no evidence of cancer, and her markers in her blood seemed to be in the normal range. There was a smile on Paul's face for the first time in months. She had planned a weekend getaway with him to celebrate away from the hustle and bustle of family life; she hoped the two of them could finally reconnect. On the drive home she reached for him and told him of her plans for the weekend. Yet Paul again rebuffed her advances; the excuses had been all used up but somehow he managed anew. This time it was a new deadline for a work project, and it had reared its head at a time that should have been full of relief and joy. The months of chemo agony were over and were now replaced with muted trepidation. With each rebuff of her advances, Shannon grew more despondent. The apprehension of her rebuffed advances plagued Shannon like the CA 125 tests that she dreaded at each visit.

It was in this state that Shannon arrived in my office. She was now one year out from completing chemotherapy treatment and was, by all measurable standards, cancer-free. Her previous cancer doctor had taken a job elsewhere, and she came in to establish care and to see what the latest research held for her cancer. I approached her care like all patients, a thorough history as well as family evaluation for cancers followed by an equally thorough physical exam. Her body had healed from the onslaught of chemotherapy and surgical attacks so common to cancer patients. Her physical exam was normal aside from the typical symptoms and signs that we see in women with gynecologic cancer. Her hair had just started to come in full, rich, and curly, as so often happens. Her skin was dry from the chemotherapy but starting to regain its normal hue.

After her exam, I told Shannon that I would recommend a chemotherapy break to see how she did and how she wanted to proceed. It was at this point that she became increasingly despondent and said, "I just don't want to live." This statement caught me off guard. One of the most rewarding parts of a cancer doctor's practice is seeing patients, riddled with cancer, present as cancer-free and healthy after months of fighting with surgery, chemo, and radiation. I was stunned by this reaction.

It was then she told me her love story: how she had met her husband and the whirlwind passionate romance that ensued. The dream wedding they had and the joy of raising their two boys together. She also told me about the complete deterioration of their marriage, the complete lack of any sexual or affectionate contact, and her own feelings of self-loathing. Shannon's most profound statement was, "I knew I would have to fight hard to beat ovarian cancer, but I didn't think cancer would cost me my marriage."

These words sadly ring true for many couples in an age of many competing interests that threaten the sanctity of intimate relationships. But perhaps no issue tests the tenets of intimate relationships more than chronic illness. And the "emperor of maladies" strains this more than most.

FOCUS ON GYNECOLOGIC CANCERS

While all cancers represent an affront to a person's sense of self-worth, certain cancers do affect intimate relationships in ways that are not expected. Cancers that affect the sexual organs can particularly affect the way in which cancer patients interact with their intimate partners; this seems an obvious conclusion, yet sadly it remains one of the least studied or least addressed issues with regard to cancer survivorship in medicine.

By definition, gynecologic cancers involve sexual and reproductive organs. Women who have cancer of the cervix, vulva, uterus, or ovaries know one thing for certain: It will affect their sexual functioning. The major questions are "How much of an effect will it have?" and "How long will the effect last?" Breast cancer also belongs in this discussion because breasts are the most visible sign of womanhood. Their absence doesn't physically affect sex or reproduction, but it can have a profound effect on both partners' perception of desirability.

Before focusing on the physical, hormonal, and psychological changes related to the gynecologic cancers, let's look very quickly at what's considered normal in terms of anatomy and hormones. Figure 1.1 illustrates the components of the female reproductive system, all of which can potentially be affected by one or more tumors.

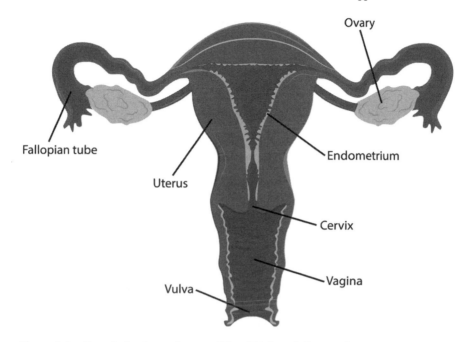

Figure 1.1. Female Anatomy. Source: ©Pavel Voinau | Dreamstime.com

In terms of sex drive and satisfaction, the ovaries are at the heart of the matter, producing the sex hormones estrogen and progesterone. Estrogen lubricates the vagina and keeps it flexible. Even when estrogen levels drop as a woman gets older, that doesn't mean the vagina has to dry up and close up; it means that changes in response to arousal may happen more slowly. The ovaries also produce some of a woman's androgens. Testosterone is the androgen we link with libido for women and men. Although ovarian hormones drop after menopause, this doesn't necessarily mean a reduction in sexual desire. The adrenal glands, which sit above the kidneys, make about half of the androgens in a woman's body, and that output can continue.

With those facts in mind, here is the good news: Even though cancer might lead to loss or alteration of body structures related to sex, and may impact hormone levels, the body has other systems and ways of coping with change that mean you can most likely have a fulfilling sex life. This book is designed to give you a clear understanding of how cancer and the treatment for it affects you, as well as the myriad paths to sexual satisfaction after you have gone through the disease and the healing.

To begin, let's consider each type of cancer individually. First, we will give an overview of changes that occur because of the cancer, and then we'll look briefly at the changes triggered by the treatment.

PHYSICAL, HORMONAL, AND PSYCHOLOGICAL CHANGES DUE TO CANCER

To introduce the discussion, we want to familiarize you with some basic terms that will recur in the book. The first set of terms is the two main types of gynecologic cancers: carcinoma and sarcoma. Carcinoma is a cancerous tumor that begins in the skin or in tissue covering an internal organ. Sarcoma is a malignancy that begins in bone, cartilage, fat, muscle, blood vessels, or other connective tissue.

The second set of terms is *invasive* and *noninvasive*. Invasive cancer means the cancer cells have broken out of the small lobe where they began. They therefore have the potential to spread to the lymph nodes, which are part of the immune system. In contrast, noninvasive cancer means those cells are contained.

The third set of terms is the stages of cancer. These stages help describe the severity of the cancer. They give a sense of how big the tumor is, the nature of it, and whether or not the cancer has spread from the original site. The National Cancer Institute provides these descriptions of the stages:[1]

Stage 0	Carcinoma in situ, which means that it is confined to its original site
Stage I, Stage II, and Stage III	Higher numbers indicate more extensive disease; larger tumor size and/or spread of the cancer beyond the organ in which it first developed to nearby lymph nodes and/or tissues or organs adjacent to the location of the primary tumor
Stage IV	The cancer has spread to distant tissues or organs

Cervical

Aisha is in her late twenties and lives in southern Africa. She exists with many names in many developing nations, but her story is the same. She works hard to help keep her family out of poverty, and so does her husband. They have two young children to whom Aisha devotes most of her free time. With a life that is almost entirely focused on the care and support of her family, Aisha ignores her own comfort and health. She dismisses intermittent vaginal bleeding, particularly after intercourse, as irregular periods. She assumes her difficulties with sex will go away; she thinks maybe she strained herself by lifting something heavy and needs time to heal.

Aisha's bleeding worsens. Soon she begins to smell. Her husband is repulsed by her, and even her children keep at a distance from her. She goes to the doctor and learns that Stage III cervical cancer is ripping through her body. It's causing fistulas, which are permanent abnormal passageways between organs or between an organ and the exterior of the body. One result: Stool is coming from her vagina, causing a horrible stench.

Women in many countries, even women in so-called developed nations, who either ignore their health or don't have access to good health care experience cervical cancer in this manner. The physical changes they endure are not only frightening for them but they can also signal the end of their marriage and their family life. The husband leaves, thinking, "I can find someone else. I can get married again." The children are too young to care for the mother or to care for themselves. A woman in rural India or Africa might simply walk into the nearest body of water and drown herself out of despair and humiliation.

Cervical cancer is the most common gynecologic cancer worldwide. It's characterized by postcoital bleeding—not a particularly romantic occurrence. The reason is that the tumor is located on the cervix, which is the lower part of the uterus, or the upper vagina; the vagina is the canal that connects the uterus to the world outside. In intercourse, the penis bangs up against the tumor. That causes bleeding and can induce a lot of pain if the nerves are impinged.

You might wonder why we say that cervical cancer is the most common worldwide but not the most common gynecological cancer in countries such as the United States and Australia. A main reason is that it's *preventable* by the human papillomavirus (HPV) vaccines that are readily available in more developed nations. And even though the vaccination rate is considered low in the United States—in 2014, only six out of ten adolescent girls had started the HPV vaccine series of three shots and only four out of ten adolescent boys had started it, according the U.S. Centers for Disease Control—in places where women like Aisha live, the rate of vaccination has been zero.[2]

The World Health Organization (WHO) notes that the mortality rate per one hundred thousand cases of cervical cancer in Australia/New Zealand, Western Asia, and Western Europe is less than 2 percent; it's just under 3 percent for the United States. That primarily reflects the availability of high-quality health care and raised awareness of symptoms. In contrast, the mortality rate in places like western and southern Africa is about 42 percent. WHO estimates that 99 percent of cervical cancer cases are linked to genital infection with HPV, which is sexually transmitted; theoretically, anyone who is not celibate or not vaccinated is at risk.

One major hormonal change that occurs with cervical cancer occurs with every cancer, gynecologic or other. It is part of experiencing fear; that is, the body's autonomic "fight or flight" biochemical response to a threat. When a human being feels fearful, cortisol levels rise and testosterone levels drop. Testosterone—often erroneously associated only with men—is a key hormone in sexual drive for both genders. A woman with cancer is nearly always a woman who is afraid; she has elevated cortisol levels and corresponding diminished sex drive.

A related change, which also applies to someone with any cancer, is a shift in dopamine levels. High dopamine levels mean you are in tune with pleasure; reduced dopamine levels mean that your perceptions of reward and pleasure are in the basement.

The psychological impact is obviously tied to the hormonal shift, but for now, let's focus on what the woman feels on learning about her cervical cancer. It depends in part on where the woman lives. That may sound odd, but someone in an environment like Aisha's would likely experience symptoms of advanced cancer so the psychological impact would be self-loathing and depression. She has become physically repulsive to the people she needs and loves most. Contrast that with a woman in the United States who gets an early diagnosis and education from her physician about the cause; that is, human papillomavirus infection. She may be angry about not having received the vaccine to prevent the cancer, angry about being infected by her partner (or a previous partner), and angry that her misfortune in those two things has led to a life-threatening disease that will end her chances of biological motherhood if she must have a hysterectomy. The one thing that may make her less angry is her chances of survival based on five-year observed survival rates recorded by the American Cancer Society:[3] In the earliest stages, her chances are greater than 90 percent and increasing all the time. Even in all of the phases considered Stage II, the chances are about 60 percent or greater.

Contrast that with what Aisha faces. Even with great care, which she is not likely to get, her chances of survival are one in three at best. And if her cancer has advanced to Stage IV, then she has about a 15 percent chance of survival.

We don't want to miss this opportunity to say that cervical cancer can nearly be eradicated if we simply inoculate our young women and our young men. The choice is simple: Get the HPV vaccine or remain celibate for the rest of your life.

Uterine/Endometrial

This is the most common cancer in the United States and Australia; one reason is that it is often linked to obesity. Not surprisingly, the United States and Australia are ranked among the fattest nations in the world. Another cause is inherited genetic predisposition.

When it's linked to obesity, a certain type of gene mutation has occurred that is acquired, or "somatic." In those cases, some time during the woman's life, mutations occurred in certain cells of the body. The cause can be environmental, as in the case of ultraviolet light triggering skin cancer or smoking causing lung cancer. With obesity, fat cells enlarge and engender additional estrogen production, thereby creating an environment that can lead to gene mutations causing uterine cancer.

The physical change is bleeding coming from a tumor growing into the wall of the uterus. Ultimately, growth of the tumor will increase the size of the uterus to the point where the woman may feel like she's pregnant. Some historians speculate that Queen Mary I (aka "Bloody Mary"), who was convinced she was pregnant in late 1557 only to die in November 1558, actually had a tumor growing in her.

Most of the time, uterine cancer hits women over fifty; the average age is sixty. Vaginal bleeding at that age, by which time most women have gone through menopause, is literally a red alert. Women with uterine cancer who are younger will have some irregularities in bleeding—perhaps a flow that contains more blood than usual—so it's important to recognize differences and get examined immediately. Other physical changes might be painful urination, painful sex, and pain in the pelvic area. In other words, if something hurts in the general area of your uterus, your body is giving you an important message.

The hormonal change in relation to fear would be the most pronounced at the point of diagnosis, although others occur later that are related to treatment. One thing that will often allay that fear is the survival rate, which is 75 percent or greater with any type of Stage I endometrial cancer. With every type of Stage II cancer, the survival rate is nearly 60 percent. Stage III has a survival rate of 50 percent or greater, according to statistics gathered by the American Cancer Society.

The main psychological impact for a young woman would be the loss of her uterus, meaning the end of any possibility of pregnancy. For older women, there might still be a sense of loss, of emptiness. Unlike the removal of an appendix, a hysterectomy means the loss of a body part that is intimately linked to her womanhood. With diagnosis comes the reality of this significant physical change.

Not everyone feels a sense of loss with a hysterectomy, though. We talked with some women over the age of fifty-five who focused on how lucky they were that their cancer was in a "container"; namely, the uterus. They weren't happy with the diagnosis, of course, but realizing that the tumor was housed in a body part they no longer needed gave them a surge of optimism.

Ovarian

Although called "rare" in the United States because there are fewer than two hundred thousand cases a year, ovarian cancer is the third most common gynecologic cancer in the United States and the most common type among women in the United Kingdom. We shouldn't actually say "it," though, because there are many variations of "it." The National Ovarian Cancer Coalition (NOCC) notes that there are more than thirty different kinds of ovarian cancer.[4] They can be grouped into three main types:

- *Epithelial*, meaning that the malignant cells are in the tissue covering the ovary. About 85 to 90 percent of ovarian cancers fall into this category. Unfortunately, it's not only the most common but also the most dangerous because symptoms don't tend to show up until the cancer has progressed.
- Malignancy in *germ cells*. These are cells in the ovary that are destined to form eggs. The NOCC notes that 90 percent of patients with this type can be cured and their fertility preserved.
- Malignancy in *stromal cells*. These are hormone-releasing cells connecting the structures of the ovaries. Tumors in these cells are rare and generally low grade, but they can recur years after initial treatment.

Among the key risk factors for ovarian cancer are a genetic predisposition and hormone replacement therapy. With the former, we are talking about mutations in the BRCA1 and BRCA2 genes (BReast CAncer susceptibility genes). These mutations are detectable through testing, so a family history of ovarian cancer signals the need to get the test. Regarding the latter, studies suggest that the risk of this cancer is higher in women who have been taking estrogen for a number of years—the American Cancer Society says at least five or ten—but not taking progesterone, the other female hormone produced by the ovaries. Other key risk factors are age and obesity, with postmenopausal women and those with a body mass index of thirty or more having a greater chance of developing ovarian cancer than their under-forty counterparts of average weight. The American Cancer Society notes that half of all ovarian cancers are found in women sixty-three years of age or older.[5]

The physical changes of the onset of ovarian cancer tend to be unnoticeable. Most pronounced manifestations of the disease present at late stage, and by that time, the cancer may have spread all over body.

For women who are sexually active, they may notice some reduction in arousal and satisfaction, since impaired ovaries mean weakened production of estrogen—and estrogen helps to lubricate the vagina. Other warning signs would be back and/or abdominal pain, unusual vaginal bleeding, nausea, and bloating. The bottom line on this or any other gynecologic cancer is that irregular vaginal bleeding and pain in your midsection should prompt you to make an appointment with your doctor immediately. Let's be blunt: Waiting is suicidal.

The ovaries have two main jobs: They produce eggs and secrete hormones. The latter function makes them an important factor in sexual arousal. In fact, you might think of the ovaries as a pleasure center—one that is underestimated and not understood by most men and women. Hopefully, this book is part of a profound transformation in that mentality.

Like testicles, a generic term for ovaries is *gonads*. All that means is that they are the primary reproductive organs. The two even look similar and develop from the same source in an embryo. In general, surgeons don't hesitate to remove ovaries—we don't see them—whereas removal of the testicles causes great consternation and alarm. But consider this: When a surgeon takes the ovaries out that is essentially castrating a woman. What's unfortunate in medicine as a whole is we have a "let's just take them out" attitude. It's a huge bias, since we would never say in a routine manner, "Let's just cut his testicles off."

Ovaries define what makes a woman a woman. The physical effects of removal, particularly for younger women, can be demoralizing.

Vulvar

This is the fourth most common gynecologic cancer. The vulva is the external part of the female genitalia. It includes the opening of the vagina; the labia, which are the outer and inner "lips" at either side of the vagina; and the clitoris. It also contains the opening of the female urethra, so it serves the essential function of passing urine. A tumor in the early stages might not cause any symptoms, but as it grows, a tumor in any of these areas would result in painful sex. And since most women don't look at this part of themselves with any regularity (or ever!), any change in appearance would be something they would probably learn from a partner. These visible changes might include white or reddish bumps, a white patch that feels rough, or an open sore that doesn't heal. The woman might also experience a burning sensation during urination or persistent itching.

Most vulvar cancer begins in squamous cells, the primary type of skin cells. Since the parts of the vulva aren't generally exposed to the sun, you might think that vulvar cancer is never melanoma or basal cell carcinoma—but that's actually not true. About six of every one hundred vulvar cancers are melanoma and, although it's very rare, sometimes vulvar cancer is basal cell.[6]

One of the causes of vulvar cancer is the same thing that causes most cases of cervical cancer; that is, the human papillomavirus. A woman exposed to HPV who also smokes increases her risk of getting vulvar cancer. (We could put this note in about smoking with the other types of cancer, too.)

The risk of developing vulvar cancer increases as a woman ages; less than 20 percent of the cases are in woman younger than age fifty. Women in the fifty to sixty age range are generally experiencing important hormonal shifts affecting their libido without the onset of disease. Knowledge that they have vulvar cancer, and awareness of what needs to be done to treat it, would likely make the libido plummet.

PHYSICAL, HORMONAL, AND PSYCHOLOGICAL CHANGES DUE TO THE TREATMENTS

All of the gynecologic cancers involve surgery because it's the logical treatment for all solid malignancies. The driving desire is to get the tumor out if possible. The common experience that women would have, regardless of the type of cancer, is the regimen of preparation, some degree of anxiety about the anesthesia and procedure, and uncertainties about how well and how quickly they will recover.

The gynecologic organs are not vital organs, but the changes that occur after removing or altering them to excise a tumor can be life altering for a woman. It's not a matter of losing an organ that puts the person's life in peril; it's a matter of losing an organ that can jeopardize quality of life because of how the woman responds biochemically and psychologically.

Every part of the female anatomy has a practical function except for the clitoris, which is solely designed for pleasure. The uterus and fallopian tubes lose their practical function after the childbearing years. But all of the other parts of the female anatomy have a job to do in supporting sexual health, among other things.

Many of the physical, hormonal, and psychological changes due to treatments are summarized in the section on cervical cancer, so regardless of your area of interest, be sure to read that section first.

Cervical

There are seven basic types of surgery for cervical cancer, and not all of them render the woman unable to have children afterward. Note that some of these types also apply to other gynecologic cancers. So even though the reason for doing the surgery is different, the procedure is the same. The seven and their immediate physical impact are:

- Cryosurgery—This can be used in cases where the cancer is not invasive. *Cryo* is a Greek prefix meaning "icy cold," so cryosurgery involves the use of cold to kill abnormal cells. The physical change most noticeable right after it is a watery-brown discharge for a few weeks.
- Laser surgery—You might think of this as the opposite of the cold approach. In laser surgery, a focused beam burns off abnormal cells or a piece of tissue. Again, this is not used to treat invasive cancer; it's a treatment for Stage 0 cancer that can be done in a physician's office.
- Conization—Different implements can be used—surgical knife, laser knife, or a heated wire—but they all accomplish the same thing: They enable the surgeon to remove a cone-shaped piece of tissue. Although this is often used as a diagnostic technique, it can also be used as a treatment for women with early stage cancer who want to preserve their ability to give birth.
- Hysterectomy—There are two types of hysterectomy, with one being more radical than the other. They both remove the uterus and cervix, but one does not take out structures next to the uterus, whereas the other one does if the surgeon determines that the cancer has spread. There are three basic ways to do a hysterectomy: removal through the abdomen, through the vagina, and by using laparoscopy. The third option involves the use of cameras and small tubes through which the surgeon removes the tissue. This is now commonly done with a robotic surgical system called DaVinci® so that the surgery is minimally invasive.
- Trachelectomy—This procedure is designed to address certain Stage I cancers in a way that still allows the woman to have children. The surgery removes the cervix and top part of the vagina, but leaves the body of the uterus intact. A band or "purse-string" stitch at the base of the uterine cavity simulates the cervical opening.
- Pelvic exenteration—This is a radical surgery involving the removal of reproductive organs and tissues as well as others in the "neighborhood." It's sometimes used to treat recurrent cervical cancer. It will be covered in greater depth in chapter 5, which features the story of a

woman with a recurrent cancer and her successful struggle not only to save her life but also her love life.

- Pelvic lymph node dissection—Sometimes, the surgeon has a concern that cancer has spread from the original site. Removal of lymph nodes while doing the hysterectomy or trachelectomy would either confirm or refute the suspicion. The immediate, uncomfortable physical result might be swollen legs since removal of the lymph nodes can lead to drainage problems in the legs.

Any surgery to remove the cervix can result in a build-up of scar tissue after surgery and cause the vaginal tube to diminish in length. Intercourse might be a bit painful after this, but as we discuss later in the book, there are ways to compensate for the change.

The latest science indicates that the loss of cervix doesn't have a dramatic impact on sexual satisfaction. The same can be said for the uterus. Unless the ovaries were removed in the surgery, the biggest biochemical response would be fear related; that is, elevated cortisol levels and reduced testosterone levels.

When chemotherapy is introduced into the treatment regimen, risk factors for sexual dysfunction increase in number. This applies no matter what gynecologic organs are involved. Chemotherapy tends to lead to some interrelated results, all of which can affect the woman's desire and ability to have a fulfilling sex life:

- Fatigue, and in fact, the patient might experience chronic fatigue syndrome
- Anemia; that is, a decrease in red blood cells
- Shortness of breath
- Damage to glandular functioning
  - Chemotherapy is a poison specially formulated to act on rapidly dividing cells. It can affect any glandular organ profoundly, irrespective of the cancer diagnosis.
  - During chemotherapy treatment, steroids are introduced to decrease the risk of the patient having an allergic reaction. Depending on the frequency and nature of the chemotherapy, the repeated exposure to these steroids could have an adverse affect on the pituitary gland, blood sugar levels, and other functions.
- Loss of hair. One of the things that define femininity for many women is their hair. Chemotherapy affects the hair follicles, and with few exceptions, when we see a woman without hair she has cancer. It's like the scarlet letter worn by Hester Prynne in Nathaniel Hawthorne's novel: People cannot help but stare. The psychological effect can be devastating.

Radiation therapy might also be used for cervical cancer, often in conjunction with chemotherapy. As in the discussion of the effects of surgery and chemotherapy, many of the comments here apply to radiation to treat other gynecologic cancers. The external beam radiation therapy (EBRT) used to treat cervical cancer is given like an X-ray, except that the radiation dose is significantly stronger. The physical effects of having EBRT can include:

- Fatigue
- Upset stomach
- Diarrhea or loose stools
- Nausea and vomiting
- Skin changes, such as temporary redness like a bad sunburn

With pelvic radiation, women lose ovarian function unless the surgeon takes precautionary action. Especially when the patient is a young woman, the surgeon might move the ovaries out of the way—almost all the way to the liver—otherwise they will shrink and die. There are also physical changes in the vagina, with the vagina shrinking and drying up. The medical term for the result is *dyspareunia*, which means that intercourse causes genital pain, and, therefore, sexual dysfunction.

Brachytherapy, which is a type of internal radiation therapy, may also be used to treat cervical cancer; it's often used in addition to EBRT. A metal cylinder filled with radioactive material is inserted in the vagina. Radiation administered in this manner travels only a very short distance and often has no immediate side effects, except perhaps a little irritation in the vaginal area. Sometimes, patients have a mild version of the other effects associated with radiation in addition to that. To prevent a serious long-term effect of brachytherapy, the patient has to keep the vaginal opening from becoming extremely narrow and inflexible. That result is called vaginal stenosis, and can be prevented by stretching the walls of the vagina regularly, especially during the first few months after the therapy. As you might imagine, either the radiation oncologist in charge of the treatment or an assistant in the practice will sit the patient down—preferably with the woman's partner—and ask the Big Question: "Do you promise to have sex several times a week, or will you be using a vaginal dilator?" Depending on the nature of the brachytherapy, some women have to stretch the walls daily and for such duration that sexual intercourse is not a viable alternative. We also need to note that the elasticity of the vagina, in addition to severe dryness, means that intercourse cannot be "business as usual."

Since brachytherapy involves a handful of people and the patient's vagina is the focus of attention, all of those medical professionals are likely to introduce themselves and explain why they are in the room. One of those people is a physicist, and that might well prompt the question: "Why is there a physicist looking at my vagina?" Among other things, the radiation physicist on the team controls the timing of the therapy—and with brachy, it could be just a couple of minutes, depending on the equipment used. In some facilities, it's the physicist who remains with the patient and keeps her informed, "Okay thirty seconds down and seventy-three seconds to go." In other facilities, there is no one in the room with the patient because the equipment being used requires all staff to be behind a protective shield.

After radiation, the glands in epithelial tissue (the tissue covering the organ) are largely dead. The place that used to be taken for granted as a pleasure center now needs help to serve that purpose each and every time that intercourse is desired. Restoration of sexual function necessitates the use of a water-based lubricant during treatment (any other is fine after treatment), and—whether with the aid of a dilator or sexual intercourse—making sure the vagina is opened regularly without force. More on this later!

Uterine/Endometrial

The primary treatment for uterine cancer is a hysterectomy, described above. If the cancer has spread to neighboring organs, then the hysterectomy is the radical version. Complementary surgeries to remove the fallopian tubes and ovaries and/or lymph nodes may be done at the same time. Again, the above section on surgeries for cervical cancer describes the immediate physical effects of the procedures.

Chemotherapy may follow the hysterectomy, but not necessarily. If so, after a brief recovery period at the completion of the chemo, the patient will have brachytherapy.

In the short term, the challenges of healing from surgery, fatigue from treatments, and so on will naturally affect a woman's desire to have sex. In the long term, after the patient has recovered from the treatments, there is no physical reason why removal of the uterus should prevent a woman from having a fulfilling sex life. And yet, as you will see in upcoming chapters, it often does.

Ovarian

A hysterectomy and removal of the fallopian tubes and ovaries is generally used when the tumor is in the ovary. But if the patient wants to retain the option to bear children, and the tumor is only in one ovary, the surgeon may remove only the affected ovary.

Symptoms of ovarian cancer don't necessarily show up until the disease has progressed, especially with the epithelial version, so it can be difficult to determine what stage it's in. Whether the tumor is in the tissue covering the ovary or in the ovary itself, the surgery has to accomplish two things: help the oncologist determine the stage of the cancer and debulk the tumor; that is, remove as much of it as possible.

In addition to the surgery, chemo might be part of the treatment, but radiation is generally not part of the regimen.

Vulvar

A 1983 study published in the *American Journal of Obstetrics and Gynecology* postulated in an opening paragraph that "mild levels of marital distress may exist (after vulvar surgery)" and quickly followed that with the note that "sexual functioning and body image appear to undergo major disruption despite the fact that intercourse remains possible." These seem like gross understatements in light of the reality, described just one paragraph later, that the surgery is "severely disfiguring."

The vaginal tube is not affected by the surgery, but in terms of appearance, the area is very different. Surgeons are aware of the cosmetic damage of the surgery, however, and take special measures to do reconstructive work, possibly even bringing in a plastic surgeon to consult. They try to spare the vagina whenever possible, but if it's removed, they will build a new one created out of skin, intestinal tissue, or muscle and skin grafts.

Chemotherapy and radiation might also be used after surgery to treat the disease.

The above was an overview of treatment options and effects, but these aren't the only ones. Biological therapy is another type of treatment, for example, that would be used in conjunction with the ones discussed. It involves the use of living organisms such as bacteria to stimulate the immune system in the fight against the cancer. Biological therapy, also referred to as immunotherapy, might be used to counter side effects of the other therapies rather than to attack the cancer itself, so they receive more attention later in the book.

We opened the chapter by noting that breast cancer deserves a place in the discussion because of the obvious way breasts help define femininity. They are the most sexual part of a woman that can be seen with her clothes on, so it's perfectly logical that removal of one or both can psychologically affect the desire to have sex. Compound that visible sign of change with others such as fatigue and hair loss from chemotherapy, and a woman may feel completely undesirable. And it's a perception that her partner may inadvertently reinforce.

Two psychological effects relate to all of the types of gynecologic cancers and breast cancer and their treatments:

- *Fear.* No matter how curable, or how treatable, the cancer is, the fear of dying is innate. Regardless of the type, there is also fear of rejection by a partner—women with gynecologic or breast cancer are more likely to be rejected by a partner. And with any treatment for gynecologic cancers, women can't have sex for a while—maybe weeks or even months. Every day, they may live with a fear of abandonment, of not being there for their partner and children.
- *Anger.* Many women resent what's happened to them: "I run every day. I eat well. I don't smoke and I drink moderately." They wonder what they could have done differently when they felt they hadn't done anything "wrong" in the first place. Science might tell them that the cause is in their genes, but they still have anger. In some cases, the anger is other-focused because the cervical or vulvar cancer resulted from HPV infection.

Changes in physical structures, hormones, and feelings are inevitable in the process that begins with diagnosis and continues with treatment. What comes next is largely mental and emotional.

It's the treating physician's job to do everything possible to help the patient deal with the physical and biochemical issues related to gynecologic cancers. But it's the patient's job—hopefully, along with her partner—to move toward complete mental health and reclaim the right to fulfillment in her most intimate relationship.

· 2 ·

What Happens Next?

$\mathcal{A}$fter the realization has set in for a woman that her life now involves a battle against cancer, she and the people around her must answer the question, "What happens next?"

Hospitals give you a three-ring binder (or envelope of papers) so that you have a handy reference on medications, red alerts, and contact numbers related to your surgery. Before chemotherapy, you get another set of papers that cover nausea, fatigue, and other possible side effects. Before radiation, you generally get another envelope. There are all kinds of answers to "What happens next?" in those documents, but you're not likely to find answers to questions like "When can I be intimate with my partner again?" "When that part of me is gone, will I still be desirable?" "Can I still enjoy sex?" "Will it feel the same?" "Do I have to do anything different when I have sex?"

The answers to these questions begin with a discussion so basic, you might think we're joking about the need for it. But there is a need for it, and you'll soon see why.

HOW SEX WORKS

Let's start with a close look at the anatomy and physiology of sex to have a common language to understand how cancer and cancer treatment affects sexual response. Hopefully, you'll find the details here that fill in missing pieces of information, from "What organ is in charge?" to "Where's that illusive G-spot?"

Anatomically, sexual response in women is a complex process that involves not only the sexual organs but also a complex series of interactions among the eyes, brain, skin, and sexual organs. A basic review of the female and male anatomy will enrich your understanding of this.

The ovaries are two small organs on either side of the pelvis that house the eggs (aka ova). They contain the cells that make the female hormone estrogen, which is involved in a host of functions in women that we will discuss later. The ovaries are attached to the uterus or womb via the fallopian tubes, the long structures that carry the egg to the uterus. The uterus itself is a thick-walled muscular organ that lies in the dead center of the pelvis. We often think of the uterus as the "muscle head" of the female reproductive system: It follows orders from the big boss, the ovaries. The ovaries send hormonal signals to the uterus to thicken its lining each month, and once those signals go away, the lining is shed though the cervix, the opening of the bottom of the uterus into the vaginal canal that receives the penis during sexual intercourse. Outside the vagina are the labia; that is, skin line folds that serve as the entrance to the vaginal canal. In between the upper part of the labia is the clitoris, the female equivalent of the penis—in actuality the tissue is nearly identical—though obviously considerably smaller.

To move on, we have to break down sex into its physiologic and hormonal processes. There are probably at least a few facts in this part of the discussion that will be new to you, primarily because this is the material in sex education class that you thought was boring—or it's the stuff that your teachers thought was "inappropriate." In a medical sense, the sexual response cycle in women can be described as three phases:

1. *Arousal.* The name is largely self-explanatory and, for women, represents perhaps the most important part of the cycle. The more commonly used term is foreplay, which is physiologically associated with several changes in the female and male body. After sexual attraction is established, blood flow to the hands and genital organs increases. The vagina, clitoris, and surrounding tissues become engorged and full of blood. The nipples and breast tissue also become engorged, and stimulation of these organs can add to female response. During the arousal phase, heart rate increases, as do breathing and blood pressure. The increase in blood pressure and heart rate contribute to the excitement of sex, similar to the anticipation that runs through a scary movie. The operative word is *anticipation*—a key element in desire. The increase in breathing rate can also create a low-level high as breathing of carbon dioxide gas quickly can actually create a slightly drowsy, quasi-awake state. As arousal continues, the face becomes increasingly flushed, and a small of amount of skin-color change can actually occur on the upper torso.

   As arousal progresses the uterus elevates and the muscles of the vagina tighten. Additionally, and most importantly for this discussion, the vagina becomes increasingly lubricated with fluid produced from the large glands surrounding it (bartholins and skenes glands). This is vital for sexual pleasure in both men and women; without appropriate lubrication, sex is almost uniformly not pleasurable for women due to the pain of the penis touching the dry vagina, and equally unpleasurable for the man. As sexual interaction progresses, a brief plateau phase is reached allowing for both the male and female sex organs to prepare for orgasm: The labia outside the vagina continue to constrict and, in men, the prostate and seminal vesicles, which assist the male orgasm, prepare appropriate fluids.

2. *Climax*, or *orgasm*. This physiologic process is vastly different in men and women. For men, the process of climax is obvious and occurs with ejaculation or release of fluid from the penis. In women, the process of orgasm is generally accompanied by rhythmic contraction of the uterus and lower vagina and release of a small amount of fluid.

   Women whose clitoris and vagina are intact have a couple of options on orgasm: clitoral and G-spot. Actually, there are a couple of others that build on the basic two, which would be a combination of the two simultaneously, and multiple orgasms. The how-to information on all of them is in part II; here we are just focused on the "where" of the clitoris and G-spot. Often described as a "bulb" or "button," the external part of the clitoris is near the vagina; the internal part extends into the vagina and heads up to the G-spot. Its sole function is pleasure, and it's well equipped to deliver it: With eight thousand nerve endings, it has twice as many as a man's penis. The G-spot is in the vagina, close to the urethra, which is why stimulation of it triggers a sense that you need to urinate—a sense that dissipates as the stimulation continues.

   Regardless of how you achieve orgasm, you will probably feel happy, or even giddy, because the experience releases endorphins into your bloodstream. These are hormones secreted within the brain and nervous system that activate opiate receptors, so they are "feel good" hormones.

3. *Resolution*. After orgasm, the heart rate slowly comes down, blood pressure decreases, and there is an overall sense of conclusion. Women may be able to orgasm again during this period, although it is very difficult for men. This is also accompanied in many women and men by intense skin and nipple sensitivity.

   The hormone *oxytocin* appears to be released during orgasm as well as hugging, touching, pregnancy, childbirth, and breastfeeding. It's often called the "love hormone," but it might be more appropriately labeled the "trust hormone." It helps to reduce stress, so it's associated with a sense of comfort, relaxation, and bonding, particularly with women. Another hormone, vasopressin, seems to have a similar effect in males.

Note that we provided the qualifying phrase in a medical sense before describing sexual response. This is because a core message of the book is that there are other legitimate ways to describe sexual response. They all involve arousal, but—surprise!—they don't all involve the genitals. They all involve satisfaction, but they don't all lead to orgasm. Making orgasm an integral part of the endgame of a sexual encounter makes sex goal oriented. Sexual intimacy is not a sport. There is no goal line, post, basket, or home plate.

One set of facts you will see presented in various ways throughout the book is how many parts of the human body are extremely sensitive to touch—and there is no practical reason they are sensitive to touch. Human females have lips, nipples, and a clitoris with an extraordinary number of nerve endings that deliver pleasure. That's all they appear to be designed to do.

The science of sex is incredibly important to a discussion about the way in which cancer affects sexual function. Cancer itself causes several alterations in the hormonal balance of a person's body. But perhaps more than the cancer itself, it is the treatment for the cancer that impacts how sexual and intimate relationships proceed. A close examination of the ways in which cancer treatment is necessary brings some key challenges into focus—with the ways to address those challenges the primary duty of the second part of this book.

PHYSICAL EFFECTS OF TREATMENTS

There are four primary ways that mainstream medical science treats gynecologic and breast cancer: surgery, radiation, chemotherapy, and immunotherapy. This is not to say that therapies such as hypnosis and massage are not embraced by mainstream medicine, but they wouldn't play a role in patient healing and comfort until later, as useful ways to address fatigue, anxiety, pain, and sleep problems, for example.

Surgery

From the dawn of time, surgery has been the mainstay by which cancer has been treated. This makes logical sense to patients. If there is a tumor, one of the simplest solutions is simply to cut it out in the hope that will make the cancer go away. For many patients this seems to be the most important means by which to cure their cancer. We know that in many early stage cancers, this is certainly the way to go. The fact remains, however, that surgery alone rarely cures cancer, and other adjuvant treatments are necessary in the form of chemotherapy or radiation, or sometimes both. Yet at the heart of treatment for solid tumors is the notion of debulking; that is, surgery to remove the tumor.

Surgery itself carries a host of changes, some of which were mentioned in chapter 1 in relation to the different gynecologic cancers. We want to be a bit more general in this section to focus on the overall experience of surgery. The immediate postoperative period is punctuated by many milestones: the groggy haze of waking up from surgery, the initial pain of the surgical wound, the pulling of the surgical staples vital to hold the skin together, and the weeks of a dull ache as the sutures holding everything together resorb. Scar tissue begins to form in just a few days after surgery, and the adhesions that are the exaggerated response to inflammation in the body also start to appear. All of these changes, and the off-and-on pains, contribute to an inhibition of sexual desire. It's a bit like having the flu—you feel off your game and know that parts of you aren't very pretty at the moment. But perhaps unique to surgery is the actual physical changes that occur when removal of organs and tumors take place.

In women afflicted with gynecologic cancer, surgery has several profound effects on the sexual organs, with some effects more pronounced than others depending on the disease site. First, cancers of the uterus and ovary almost always require removal of both ovaries. The ovaries not only house the eggs that are required for reproduction, but they are also filled with rich supporting cells that make estrogen, the female hormone. Estrogen has myriad functions and is critical in the sexual response process. With surgical removal of the ovaries (surgical menopause), there is a host of changes in the female sexual cycle. In addition to serving as an estrogen source, the ovaries are a powerhouse of other hormones, responsible for making nearly 30 percent of a woman's circulating testosterone. Testosterone is mainly thought of as a male hormone, but it has as key role in sexual drive, or libido, in women. In fact, it's required for a satisfying sexual life in the conventional sense of aiming for orgasm. This is another reason why surgical removal of the ovaries tends to severely inhibit a woman's sex drive. Since 70 percent of a women's estrogen is made in the ovaries, removal of them results in an instant menopause and associated symptoms such as hot flashes, irritability, impaired libido, and vaginal dryness. Without estrogen to stimulate the glands of the vagina to produce fluid, intercourse can be painful. Additionally, estrogen causes increased blood flow to the clitoris and labia so that when they are stimulated, sexual response is enhanced.

Surgical removal of the ovaries can also cause scar tissue to form at the site where the ovaries resided as well as at the top of the vagina if the patient has had her uterus and cervix removed. This scar tissue can lead to pain in the pelvis that sexual activity might exacerbate. Many women complain that sexual intercourse can be painful after surgical removal of the ovaries even when they are on hormone replacement therapy.

Removal of the breasts can also profoundly affect both sexual desire and pleasure. There are two main surgical procedures that women with breast cancer undergo that affect the breast: mastectomy (removal of the entire breast) and lumpectomy (removal of a small portion of the breast). Breast tissue itself, particularly the area around the nipple, is one of the innervated parts of the body and is among the more erogenous zones on the body for many people. This is true for both women and men, so disruption of this area can affect sexual functioning in both physical and psychological ways.

From a physical perspective, stimulation of the breasts often causes a cascade of events in the female body that is vital to pleasure for women. Once the breasts and nipples have been stimulated, a series of hormonal signals causes the breasts themselves to become engorged and larger. These hormonal changes cause an increase in blood flow to the labia, vagina, and clitoris, further enhancing sexual responsiveness. Surgery on the breasts, including breast augmentation surgery, can cause nerve damage around the nipple that can inhibit these important hormonal signals.

Nipple preservation surgery becomes exceedingly important to this process and should be discussed with the operating surgeon. This is not to say that it maintains sensation—that does not seem to be the case—but because it contributes to a more natural postimplant appearance. After actress/activist Angelina Jolie had her preventative double mastectomy, breast surgery that keeps the nipple and surrounding skin intact became popularly known as "Angelina Jolie–style surgery." Some women we spoke with enjoyed the cosmetic advantage that this type of surgery gave them; others arrived at a different option with their plastic surgeon.

From a psychological perspective, surgical removal of the breasts is arguably among the most disfiguring surgeries in cancer care. For many women, more than any other organ, breasts define a woman's sense of femininity, attractiveness, and womanhood. They are a source of pride, and society and the media have deemed the breasts as the defining aspect of a woman's physique. Even though the ovaries are more essential to sexual functioning, no one sees photos of ovaries in a bikini.

This focus on the psychological aspects of cancer surgery points to an incredible difference between how men and women are often treated by their doctors. Physicians tend to remove the ovaries and breasts with a certain laissez-faire indifference: If they house disease, the solution is to remove them. Yet this is not the same for men. The tendency is almost never to remove the testicles unless absolutely necessary, and almost all men with testicular cancer are fitted with a prosthesis to ensure aesthetics and symmetry of the gonadal area. For women, ovaries and breasts are removed far more quickly—sadly without thought about the potentially huge psychological implications.

Breast cancer awareness is changing this bias, as is the growing number of women in surgical roles.

Radiation

One the most important steps in the armamentarium of cancer treatment is the use of radiation to treat cancers. Radiation therapy works by sending radioactive particles into tissue—specifically fast-dividing tissue like cancer—with the goal to kill it at the molecular level. This therapy has evolved dramatically over the last one hundred years and continues to be a mainstay with regard to cancer treatment and therapy. In many cancers such as breast and cervical cancer, cure rates with radiation therapy are very high, particularly in early stage disease. In fact, cure rates with regard to cervical cancer are as good as surgery in many cases. Radiation is mainly used in what we call the adjuvant setting; that is, after surgery has removed the majority of the cancer, radiation is then used to sterilize the residual or microscopic disease. This is used most frequently in breast, uterine, and cervical cancer. Radiation itself is not something that patients necessarily feel "going in," and it's administered by a radiation oncologist, a physician who specializes in this therapy.

Radiation is not without its impact on sexual functioning. Radiation particles, which mostly target cancer cells, can also have an effect on normal tissue as well. The lining of the vagina, bladder, and rectum are particularly sensitive to radiation therapies. After radiation is administered, these tissues undergo some degree of atrophy, or weakening. Particularly sensitive to this are the glands in the vagina that make the canal itself wet and ultimately pleasurable for sexual intercourse. As these glands are further exposed to radiation, the ability to produce the fluid that lubricates the vagina during the arousal phase of intercourse becomes further impaired. As a result, after several weeks of radiation treatment, the vagina becomes dry and sexual relations can become increasingly painful. The bladder and rectum are also susceptible to these changes, and a small amount of blood (cystitis) can be seen during urination as well as pain with bowel movements (prostatic). Another very common side effect after treatment of the pelvic area with radiation is the development of vaginal stenosis or shortening/narrowing of the vaginal canal itself. One of the unique properties of the vaginal canal is its inherent lack of rigidity and ability to expand and slightly dilate with sexual activity; this elasticity allows sex to be pleasurable for both men and women. During radiation therapy, this elastic ability of the vagina to expand becomes impaired as a side effect of the treatment. This can result in painful relations, particularly at the time of insertion as the vagina has become increasingly rigid. It's distressing not only for women but also for men since a partner screaming in pain does little to stimulate sexual activity. Fortunately, there are very effective measures that can be taken to mitigate stenosis and counter the dryness problem, and they are addressed in depth in part II. These are postradiation "requirements" generally covered in a briefing that a female physician's assistant or nurse in the radiation oncologist practice gives to the woman and, in some radiation oncology practices, to her partner.

Radiation causes another side effect that will diminish a woman's interest in having sex: fatigue. The body uses a lot of energy to fight the cancer cells and rebuild healthy cells; compound that stress with blasts of radiation or chemotherapy, and you can end up with a very tired and weak woman. Interestingly, fatigue may not set in right away; in fact, it often doesn't hit with full force until two or three weeks after radiation treatment. Even after completing treatment, it generally takes a month or more for a person's energy level to return to normal.

Chemotherapy

Perhaps the most dreaded part of cancer treatment for women is chemotherapy. The first reaction to this that we see with so many patients is one of agony, horror, and despair. Visions of heads over the toilet vomiting, hair loss, and extreme fatigue are the first things that come to mind when the c word—it doesn't just stand for *cancer*—is mentioned.

We should interject here, for those who are relatively new to the subject, that modern science has come a long, long way since chemotherapy was first used in the early part of the twentieth century. The medicines used in infusions are calibrated, balanced, and administered in ways to reduce discomfort. And as you will learn in part II, there are specific, effective ways to avert the most dreaded side effects of chemo.

Chemotherapy works by inhibiting the growth and division of cancer cells usually through inhibiting the DNA replication process. Chemo is generally attracted to cells that are rapidly dividing, as cancer cells do; as a result the treatments tend to affect mainly cancer cells and leave normal ones alone. However, there are a few cells in the body that are also rapidly dividing—hair follicles being one. As a result, some cancer treatments deposit in these areas and cause some of the stigma of cancer treatment. Another area that chemo wreaks havoc on is the immune system, particularly the bone marrow. Cancer patients are more susceptible to infection because chemotherapy affects the rapidly dividing cells of the bone marrow. White blood cells, which help fight off infection, and red blood cells, which deliver oxygen to tissues, are particularly susceptible to the ill effects of chemotherapy.

Chemotherapy affects sexual functioning in a variety of ways. Perhaps the most direct way is by inducing a fairly profound fatigue in patients, and the level of fatigue generally seems to be greater in women than men. Many chemotherapy agents induce a profound anemia or decrease in the red blood cell count. Red blood cells are the principal way that oxygen gets from the lungs to the tissues throughout the body and is vital for cells to work properly. As red blood cell counts decrease, so does the ability of tissue to receive oxygen and, as a result, patients feel weak. People with low energy are likely to have low sexual desire, of course. Reaching orgasm in these states also becomes more and more difficult as the oxygen need for the sexual organs to work properly becomes further impaired.

Another physical effect with psychological repercussions is hair loss. The loss of hair represents a unique phenomenon for women with cancer. For men, hair loss is a dreaded, yet in many ways an expected, event in a man's life. It doesn't necessarily make it any easier, but genetics have helped manage a man's expectations. For women, hair is at the heart of the definition of womanhood. Many women will readily admit that the part of their daily cosmetic routine that consumes the most time is upkeep and presentation of their hair. Hair and hairstyles go a long way toward defining the sexuality of a woman—straight or gay. For men, a woman's hair is also important. It attracts them on a basic level and is very much a part of the courting process. It follows, then, that hair loss can translate into a lack of feminine identity. There may be no more painful a sign that a woman has cancer than a bald head. Additionally, the immediate visceral response to a woman with no hair is that she is sickly or uninviting. There could be no more hurtful commentary to womanhood—or personhood—than that.

Another element of appearance that might change with cancer treatment is weight gain or loss. In the period immediately after surgery, many women will lose a significant amount of weight; this is true for both abdominal surgery as well as breast surgery. This weight loss occurs for a few reasons. One is that shifts in body fluids cause women to swell initially after surgery, and then the fluid is slowly lost as urine. Another reason for weight loss is decreased appetite after surgery and general feelings of malaise, with the result that patients simply just don't have an appetite. While appealing to many patients, rapid, unintentional weight loss itself is associated with a slew of issues in patients. Skin that had been stretched out due to being overweight may now have unsightly stretch marks. Weight gain is also not uncommon in women after surgery for gynecologic and breast cancer. This is mainly the result of the drugs that are used to prevent allergic reactions and complications of chemotherapy—steroids. Steroids are used oftentimes to prevent an exaggerated response to the body of chemotherapy as well as to prevent intense nausea and vomiting. Steroids can be profound appetite stimulants and cause a host of metabolic changes that promote weight gain, increase blood sugar levels, increase water retention, and promote swelling of the face, arms, and legs.

Immunotherapy

Immunotherapy is a relatively new addition to the ammunition to attack gynecologic and breast cancers, and it might be used in conjunction with some or all of the other treatments already described. The premise of it is that the white blood cells in the body called T-cells are like soldiers when it comes to disease. They patrol the body looking for signs of the "enemy"; that is, infections. They have specialized protein receptors that allow them to distinguish between normal cells and cancerous ones. When they make a positive identification that they've made contact with a cancerous cell, they launch an attack to destroy it. But cancer cells aren't stupid. Some can mask their presence with so-called checkpoint proteins that make them undetectable to T-cells. One particular disguising protein that might be used is called PD-L1, which would "mate" with the T-cell's PD-1 protein, thus convincing the T-cell that all's well. The T-cell then leaves the cancer cell alone and allows it to replicate unabated. The success of immunotherapy is grounded in the ability to block that PD-L1 "mating" with PD-1. The therapy relies on human antibodies to essentially come between the two types of protein; that allows the T-cell to do its job.

As we said, the use of immunotherapy in the types of cancers we're discussing here is relatively new. For example, the first paper documenting the clear benefits of Herceptin in treating breast cancer was published in the *Journal of Clinical Oncology* on June 1, 2010.[1] Herceptin fights breast cancer called HER2+ (*H*uman *E*pidermal growth factor *R*eceptor 2-positive), and it's used in early stage treatment.

Side effects of this and other immunotherapy can be fever and chills, nausea, vomiting, pain, shortness of breath, and even more serious health issues such as heart problems. In that sense, it isn't necessarily "better" than chemo even though it sounds more natural because it's putting the body's own T-cells to work. In fact, the Dana-Farber Cancer Institute—research home of Gordon Freeman, PhD, the "father of PD-L1"—says this about immunotherapy:

> The drugs don't directly assault the cells; instead, they free the patient's own defensive forces to destroy cancers.
>
> But it's a two-edged sword. Freed from checkpoint restraint, the surging immune response can overshoot its target and attack healthy tissues and organs, similar to an autoimmune disorder.[2]

So, even though the dreaded side effect of hair loss doesn't occur, the other chemolike effects cited above can occur. And because there is the possibility of an overactive immune response causing problems, patients would have to be monitored for things such as skin rashes, colitis, and lung inflammation.

In terms of its impact on sexual functioning, we would just say that, with the exception of hair loss, just about everything that applies to chemo applies to immunotherapy.

PSYCHOLOGICAL/EMOTIONAL EFFECTS OF TREATMENTS

All of the physical changes described above can profoundly affect body image, energy, and sensation, thereby inhibiting sexual desire.

Now consider this: A woman facing a hysterectomy, mastectomy, or any other surgery related to her cancer, is facing an empty space. Some part of her body related to her reproductive or nurturing systems will be removed. How's that for a blow to the libido? Add to that the effects of treatment such as fatigue, hair loss, dry and possibly discolored skin, a dry vagina, vomiting, and scars. It's no wonder, then, that likely psychological outcomes are the psychological Siamese twins of embarrassment and low self-esteem.

You're wearing your wig and some makeup. You look in the mirror and think, "No one would know. I look perfectly normal." That's exactly what Shelly thought when she had guests over for wine and cheese about a month after she finished her series of chemo treatments. When her guests left—she found this out later—Sarah said to Bill, "She has cancer." Sarah had been an oncology nurse, so she'd had ample exposure to the effects of chemo on skin. She recognized the pale, dry skin as one set of changes that can occur after chemo. Some people experience dryness and hyperpigmentation, or darkening of the skin. Still others develop flushing or rashes. Photosensitivity is common, so going to the beach means lots of sunscreen, cover-ups, and umbrellas.

When you realize that other people might be seeing changes that you aren't aware of, or have gotten accustomed to so they are no longer apparent to you, that can fuel the embarrassment inherent in your whole cancer experience.

A year after their visit to her house, Shelly visited Sarah and Bill and spent a lot of time outdoors at their home by the water. Thinking nothing of periodic exposure to midday sun—she'd always handled sun exposure very well, generally tanning easily—Shelly experienced unprecedented photosensitivity. Sarah let her know that the effects of chemo can last a long time, depending on the type of chemo; it was the same message she'd received from the hair stylist who "rehabilitated" her hair after it grew out. He said, "Don't expect it to be perfectly normal for two years."

Like a lot of cancer patients, Shelly figured she was cured and moved on, not absorbing the wisdom of people like her stylist. Giving yourself time to completely get over the cancer and the treatments is part of what's required to mitigate the emotional effects of them. That includes taking precautions to prevent things such as dryness and sunburn.

Let's make the matter of embarrassment over appearance even worse and consider that, although many people with cancer have insurance, insurance rarely pays for everything related to treatment. For the rest of the population, cancer involves a great many out-of-pocket expenses, so resources that might have gone to a new dress or great hairstylist—something to make the patient feel a little more attractive—aren't there. Much of the guidance we include in the second half of the book is centered on affordable or even no-cost ways to address sexual dysfunction. These are the not-so-little "little things" that can make the difference between sadness over feeling sexually undesirable and excitement over doing something that leads to satisfaction.

So after you've faced the realities of embarrassment and limited resources, you think, "I've been beaten up enough! What more could go wrong?" The answer is this: ignorance about what constitutes sexual dysfunction. It's a matter of not being able to put your finger on the issues and answers related to changes in your sexual intimacy. Getting a grasp of those issues and answers is the major point of chapter 3.

· 3 ·

Issues and Some Answers

$\mathcal{A}$s part of the gynecologic oncology practice at the University of Colorado School of Medicine, we designed and led a groundbreaking study, completed in 2015, called "Sexual & Marital Dysfunction in Women with Gynecologic Cancer." The study is as unique as the funding source for it. The Patty Brisben Foundation directs resources solely toward research on women's sexual health and is funded by the founder of Pure Romance, the world's leading woman-to-woman direct seller of relationship-enhancement products. The purpose of the study was to put issues related to gynecologic cancer patients and sexual functioning front and center and to unearth some answers that could help other women—and their partners—rediscover and sustain intimacy. It was groundbreaking because no study to date had examined in great detail the effect that gynecologic cancer has on marital and domestic partner relationships.

At the time, the preponderance of studies related to sexual functioning after cancer focused on men, such as the Livestrong Foundation survey of 3,100 cancer survivors in 2010. Other than that, there was one U.S.-based study published in 1998 on "Life after Breast Cancer: Understanding Women's Health-Related Quality of Life and Sexual Functioning,"[1] and another in 2009 on "Quality of Life and Sexual Functioning after Cervical Cancer Treatment: A Long-Term Follow-Up Study."[2] A European team contributed "Sexual Dysfunction and Infertility as Late Effects of Cancer Treatment" in 2014.[3]

Although we are going to weave in relevant findings from many published studies in this chapter and those that follow, the focus here is on the current, enlightening findings of the UC study.

ISSUES IN A STUDY ON SEXUAL DYSFUNCTION

In terms of study design and participation, the main things to know about the UC study are these:

- The study had two primary aims: to investigate a significant decline in a woman's sexual function from prediagnosis to posttreatment for gynecological cancers and to explore how a decline in sexual function posttreatment is associated with a change in a woman's marital relationship and well-being.
- Led by Saketh Guntupalli, a professor at the University of Colorado, principal investigators were physicians at four locations: University of Colorado Denver, Denver Health Medical Center, Loma Linda University Medical Center (California), and Columbia University Medical Center (New York).
- This was a cross-sectional study, meaning that it is a type of observational study involving analysis of data collection for a distinct population at a specific point in time.
  - o Participants answered 188 questions that encompassed precancer and posttreatment experiences, and they could choose to do this online or in person. Of those 181 questions, 19 pertained specifically to sexual function; this section was called the Female Sexual Function Index (FSFI). Another subset was the Intimate Bond Measure (IBM), which was a twenty-four-question survey used to measure aspects of the patient's relationship with her partner.
  - o Women with sexual dysfunction after cancer were compared to women who reported no sexual dysfunction using paired t-tests and chi-square tests. These are tests of statistical significance; that is, they illuminate whether or not your study results occurred by random chance.
    - ▪ A t-test indicates whether or not the difference between two groups' averages probably reflects a true difference in the population from which the groups came. Let's say you ask five women who've had breast cancer and report sexual dysfunction how many times a month they have sex and they say, "An average of six times a month." Then you ask five other recent breast cancer survivors who report sexual dysfunction how many times a month and they say, "An average of twice a month." That doesn't mean much since the sample is so small. But you keep at it and, at some

point, you have three hundred women who fit the profile and report no sexual dysfunction and are having sex six times a month, and another three hundred women who report sexual dysfunction and are having sex twice a month. Now you can see the t-test in action. That sample size gives you a sense of the statistical significance of the responses.

- The chi-square (pronounced kīskwer) test is another view of what constitutes a statistically significant result. It's used to compare expected data with collected data. If there is a big difference, then you can conclude that something noteworthy happened and the question becomes, "What's causing such a significant change?" For example, you have a hypothesis that half of the six hundred recent breast cancer survivors in your survey might have experienced sexual dysfunction and half will report normal sexual functioning. That puts your study participants into one of two categories: Either they did experience sexual dysfunction or they didn't. After you administer your questionnaire, you are surprised to find out that five hundred self-report sexual dysfunction and only one hundred say that their sex life is normal. You follow the chi-square formula, go to a chart, and find out that the probability (p) of this occurring randomly is very low. You can then conclude that your hypothesis was flawed and you have statistically significant data to support a new hypothesis: that there is a causal relationship between the recent experience of breast cancer and sexual dysfunction.

• The one thousand women recruited were patients between January 15, 2014, and February 28, 2015; 328 of them completed the survey.

   ○ About one-third of the patients were in the surveillance phase of their cancer experience; that is, they had gone through the acute stage of active treatment and were now being monitored for continued health.

   ○ Women were between twenty-three and eighty-four years of age, and all had some form of gynecologic cancer: 40 percent had uterine/endometrial; 37 percent had ovarian; 13 percent had cervical; and 10 percent had another, such as vaginal or vulvar.

   The percentages are not too different from the American Cancer Society's numbers on the total number of gynecologic cancers in the United States. Using the number of cases in 2015 as the foundation for the numbers, they turn out to be as follows: 55 percent for uterine/endometrial; 22 percent for ovarian; 13 percent for cervical; and 9 percent for vaginal and vulvar. One reason for the higher percentage of ovarian patients at the centers participating in the study is likely due to the reputation of the hospitals and gynecologic oncology teams: Because ovarian cancer is generally not detected until it's advanced, the patient is likely to be referred to "state of the art" treatment whenever possible.

o The average age of participants was fifty-six years old.
o Among the participants, 57 percent were Stage I or II and 43 percent were Stage III or IV.

Now, let's step back from those specifics and take a look at the kinds of surveys and tests that might shape a study like this. Those described below were not part of the University of Colorado study, but they provide some interesting perspectives on what other researchers have used to evaluate sexual function. Most of them are relatively short and readily available online; we provide links to available surveys in the notes if you'd like to explore them. In contrast to these instruments, the University of Colorado study took about thirty minutes—generally more than twice as long as some of the others described below that incorporate relevant information about sexual dysfunction

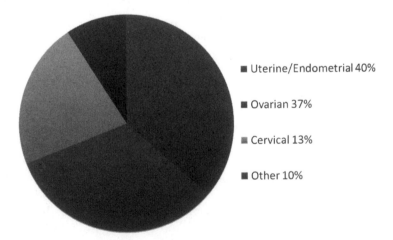

Figure 3.1.   Types of Cancer. *Note:* **57 percent were Stage I or II; 43 percent were Stage III or IV.**

but don't cover it in depth. In addition, the UC study was the first to focus on the experiences of patients across all gynecologic cancers.

- RAND Corporation is a research organization that developed a "36-Item Short Form Survey"[4] to help measure quality-of-life factors for patients. The survey asks questions about vigorous activities, such as sports, as well as moderate activities, such as carrying groceries. But these questions are precursors to focusing on issues related to social activities, pain, energy, and emotional problems that could interfere with social activities. Sex and intimacy are not mentioned specifically, but it's easy to surmise that someone who is in pain and has no energy might be asked some follow-on questions about sexual dysfunction. This is one of the survey instruments that was integral to the 1998 "Life after Breast Cancer" study, published by the American Society of Clinical Oncology, that involved 864 breast cancer survivors.
- Another instrument that figured into that study was the Centers for Epidemiologic Studies-Depression Scale (CES-D).[5] The CESD-R, which is the revised version of the screening test for depression and depressive disorder, measures symptoms defined by the *Diagnostic and Statistical Manual* (DSM) published by the American Psychiatric Association and used broadly by mental health professionals. The screening test is just twenty questions, but their focus on guilt, fatigue, sleep, movement, appetite, and interest in daily activities suggest whether or not depression might be a problem for you. The direct relevance is that depression is part of the profile of someone who's dealing with sexual dysfunction—and feels bad that she's dealing with it.
- The Dyadic Adjustment Scale (DAS) is described as a self-report measure of relationship adjustment by Multi-Health Systems, which holds the rights to it.[6] It contains thirty-two items and generally takes less than ten minutes to complete, so it's short—like the other two test instruments mentioned above. The difference is that the DAS is used with couples, so it measures both partners' perceptions. In a clinical environment, couples can learn where their ratings are different to improve their understanding of where their problems are rooted.
- The Watts Sexual Functioning Questionnaire (WSFQ)[7] is also short: a total of eleven questions for women and nineteen for men, and that includes four "both" questions. There is a big caveat with this instrument, however. If you were not sexually active within the week

prior to completing the questionnaire, then you don't qualify as a test subject. Yet if you remove the qualifying phrase *during the past week* from the questions, then the WSFQ is useful for anyone. It is a self-reporting mechanism about your ability to enjoy sex, level of desire and ease of arousal, as well as mechanical questions related to things such as lubrication and ejaculation.

- The Cancer Rehabilitation Evaluation System (CARES) comes in a long version and a short one, with subsections for people in significant relationships and people who are dating. The original author is psychologist C. Anne Coscarelli (Schag), who also published four papers in the early 1990s on the psychological and social impacts of breast cancer on survivors.[8] The papers were published within five years of publishing CARES—and obviously putting it to work. The relationship and intimacy questions, which are about both emotions and the physical aspects of having sex, are answered on a zero-to-four scale, with zero meaning "not at all" and four indicating "very much." Interestingly, with the CARES forms, the patient completing it is asked at the end of each question "Do you want help?" with the patient asked to circle Y or N. In that way, it goes beyond data collection to focus on specific needs of the individual patient.

With these studies in mind, in order for the University of Colorado study to achieve its two primary aims, participants needed to answer questions that are physical, psychological, and emotional in nature.

- The first thirteen questions collected demographic data and ended with the yes-or-no question, "Do you have any children?"
- Six questions followed that focused solely on the gynecological cancer diagnosis: the type of cancer, stage, treatments already experienced, age when diagnosed, effect of treatments on menstrual cycles (if applicable), and whether or not the patient had any other cancer diagnosis prior to the gynecological cancer.
- The eight questions that followed provided an overview of the study participants' marital or other domestic relationship.
- The next section is the first of several that's critical to establishing a baseline for further queries on sexual health because all five topics relate to feelings and behavior before the diagnosis and treatment of gynecologic cancer. With each of the statements posed, the range of seven multiple-choice answers was the degree to which it was true. For example, the statement "Before my diagnosis of cancer, sexual relations was pleasurable for me" is followed by these choices: very

strongly disagree, strongly disagree, mildly disagree, neutral, mildly agree, strongly agree, very strongly agree.
- Thirty-four more baseline questions follow in the next section. They all address problems and situations that were in place prior to cancer, such as such as feelings of frustration, anxiety, or fear related to the woman's sex life, and the degree to which she could rely on friends and her partner for moral support. There are also lots of questions related to sexual satisfaction and frequency—all tied to the relationship as it existed prior to the cancer diagnosis.

Next in the study instrument is the Intimate Bond Measure. The twenty-four questions in this section are, again, to help establish a baseline for what was normal prior to the diagnosis, and they pertain only to participants who were in a relationship with a "significant other or partner" in the weeks prior to the diagnosis. We want to note that these questions apply equally to same-sex couples and heterosexual couples and are worded to be inclusive of both types of relationships. Take a look at the first three so you get a feel for the kind of nuances that this section captures:

My partner in the weeks before my diagnosis was:

Very considerate of me:
Very True
Moderately True
Somewhat True
Not True at All

Wants me to take his/her side in an argument:
Very True
Moderately True
Somewhat True
Not True at All

Wants to know exactly what I'm doing and where I am:
Very True
Moderately True
Somewhat True
Not True at All

- After the IBM, nineteen questions compose the Female Sexual Function Index. The baselining continues here, but in this section, the questions are explicitly about desire, arousal, and so on in the four weeks before the cancer diagnosis. Here is a sampling:

In the four weeks before your diagnosis, when you had sexual stimulation or intercourse, how often did you reach orgasm (climax)?
No sexual activity
Almost always or always
Most times (more than half the time)
Sometimes (about half the time)
A few times (less than half the time)
Almost never or never

In the four weeks before your diagnosis, how often did you become lubricated ("wet") during sexual activity or intercourse?
No sexual activity
Almost always or always
Most times (more than half the time)
Sometimes (about half the time)
A few times (less than half the time)
Almost never or never

In the four weeks before your diagnosis, how often did you experience discomfort or pain during vaginal penetration?
Did not attempt intercourse
Almost always or always
Most times (more than half the time)
Sometimes (about half the time)
A few times (less than half the time)
Almost never or never

- At this point the study questionnaire is a little more than 50 percent over, and all of the remaining questions relate to the time since beginning or completion of treatment for cancer. In addition to the questions that parallel those in the sections on prediagnosis feelings and behaviors, there are those that seek the bottomline impact of cancer and treatments on the relationship:

After my diagnosis/treatment of cancer, my partner committed infidelity (had an affair).
Yes
No

After my diagnosis of cancer, my partner and I began to have significant problems in our relationship.
Very Strongly Disagree
Strongly Disagree
Mildly Disagree
Neutral
Mildly Agree
Strongly Agree
Very Strongly Agree

After my diagnosis of cancer, my partner and I needed to seek counseling/therapy to help our relationship.
Yes
No

After my diagnosis of cancer, my partner and I separated for a period of time.
Yes
No

After my diagnosis/treatment of cancer, my partner and I divorced.
Yes
No

If you've ever taken a test like the Myers-Briggs Personality Types (MBTI), you know that some of the questions seem repetitive. For example, you might check a box indicating that you strongly agree that you are a natural improviser rather than a careful planner, but later in the survey you aren't quite as committed when asked if you would rather improvise than spend time coming up with a detailed plan. The questions are not identical, but it's logical to assume that the answers would be complementary rather than contradictory. Similarly, in the UC study, some of the questions seem repetitive, but they are simply exploring the same topic from slightly different angles to get the most accurate picture of the participant's intimate relationship before and after cancer diagnosis and treatment.

ANSWERS IN A STUDY ON SEXUAL DYSFUNCTION

Consider the study results with this in mind: One of the primary reasons for marital discord as a result of a cancer diagnosis is anxiety. This seems incredibly obvious, but what may come as a surprise is that many couples experience the greatest anxiety after they've essentially beaten the cancer.

A cancer diagnosis is among the most difficult challenges that a couple will face. Some will approach it with gusto and strength—"We will beat this together!" For others, particularly those with baseline intimacy issues, the diagnosis can be the catalyst to end the relationship. They might even stick together during treatments but cancer was a big push to send the relationship off the cliff.

The anxiety factor that undermines relationships has two lives: one in the "acute" phase and one in the posttreatment, or surveillance, phase. In the acute phase, the anxiety shows up as anger ("Why did this happen to us?"), fear ("Is she going to die?"), and confusion ("How will this affect our life?"). But perhaps the most significant question—the one that few partners will admit because it sounds selfish, but it comes up in many patient interviews—is "Am I going to be left alone?" or as a corollary, "Am I going to be left alone with the kids?" When someone we love faces a crisis, we do our best to put her first and stand with her as she goes through the challenge. Yet cancer has a reputation as a thief. It steals the life and quality of life of those we love. No one wants to be robbed because it's a violation. So it's perfectly normal for a partner to feel just as violated as the cancer patient—and to ask "selfish" questions.

These questions don't necessarily linger, however. They tend to surface at the time of diagnosis and present during the acute phase of the cancer experience. Getting past the treatment phase of the experience and moving into the check-up phase answers the questions with "no" and "no," at least for the foreseeable future. Then a new anxiety comes to life, and it's one that can show up periodically, or even daily, for years to come.

This chronic anxiety isn't linked to the single goal of beating the cancer and putting it into remission. It isn't mitigated by a "fight hard" attitude. During the surveillance phase of a couple's experience of cancer, myriad insecurities, fears, and concerns can percolate to the surface, much like a tea kettle that is lukewarm that is suddenly placed on a hot burner. Think about how killers have been described many times: kept to himself, kind of quiet, and then *all of a sudden* he exploded with rage. It wasn't as though the traits that helped the rage take shape were new in his life—he was probably plagued by paranoia and low self-esteem since childhood. But something triggered a need to express the rage violently at a given moment in time. Maybe it was the loss of a job or the loss of a girlfriend.

It sounds like an extreme comparison, but for a couple going through the cancer experience, suddenly there is a triggering event: The fight is officially over. The patient has no more chemo or radiation appointments. All that's left is follow-up visits with the doctor every three months for a couple of years, and then every six months, and then maybe once a year.

This can lead to a host of psychological and emotional issues, one of which is feelings of a lack of control. Whereas before, the couple had a few three-ring binders that told them what to do, what to expect, what meds were needed—how to fight—now they have no action plan. Many patients request interventions and tests during this phase that may not serve any purpose in catching recurrent cancer. They just want to be "doing something." It's a common and disruptive way that the anxiety of the chronic phase of the experience surfaces.

With these two phases and their associated brands of anxiety in mind, take a look at the survey results, which were statistically significant in a number of key areas.

First of all, we found that sex was less pleasurable for women after cancer and that all types of sexual activity—oral, vaginal, and anal—decreased after cancer. The probability (p) that this pair of results was random was incredibly low. Both earned a value of $p > 0.001$—less than one in a thousand chance of being wrong—which is considered "statistically highly significant."

Women who reported significant sexual dysfunction following diagnosis and treatment generally fit this profile:

- Under fifty years old
- Premenopausal
- Received chemotherapy
- In a significant relationship

Looking at this profile factor by factor, we should note that older women are more likely to report less sexual activity as part of their precancer baseline than premenopausal women under the age of fifty. The contrast between precancer and postcancer numbers would therefore tend to be more dramatic for younger women. Particularly if they haven't reached menopause, they may have no dryness issues; arousal and satisfaction are relatively easy to achieve. This doesn't mean that couples in their sixties, seventies, and eighties can't have a good time, of course, but generally speaking, they slow down a bit in terms of the frequency of sexual activity.

The third bullet points to a hugely significant risk factor: chemotherapy. Women who have surgery may have obvious physical reasons why they can't resume a normal sex life for while, and even radiation can cause physical issues that need to be addressed before a normal sex life is even possible. But aside from causing relatively short-lived fatigue, and possibly a touch of nausea and bad breath—all of which can be mitigated—chemo doesn't change the body in a way that "should" lead to sexual dysfunction. But it almost invariably does.

There's just something about chemo that is profoundly disruptive for a lot of couples. One reason may be that chemotherapy has a stigma attached to it.

Many people hear the word and automatically think "horrible treatment for a deadly illness," so when they see a person they know is going through the treatment, they look for signs of deterioration. It's not as though they want the person to look horrible; they just can't stop themselves from scanning for the signs. Candy was a patient we spoke with who did not lose her hair during her series of chemotherapy sessions. She drove herself to her sessions and said she felt as though the whole experience became rather routine. And yet she felt that people around her, including her husband, treated her a little differently. Chemo was a whispered word—not something you would utter in a social situation or at the dinner table. Her husband felt reluctant to touch her. For all those reasons, she described her relatively inoffensive experience of chemo as "disgusting."

There are also self-esteem issues for a lot of women related to being visibly "damaged" by chemotherapy in the form of hair loss. Medical papers have explored topics such as "experience of patients with chemotherapy-induced alopecia," which is the technical name for partial or complete baldness. But perhaps one of the most palatable pieces on the Internet on this issue is a YouTube video called "The Stigma of Hair Loss during Chemotherapy" by a bald young woman named Sarah. She takes viewers on a seven-minute, fifty-six-second journey from hair loss and sorrow to a new vision of herself. If every woman who loses her hair could go through this journey to the end, chemo might be "put in its place" instead of given so much power to ruin a woman's life for a while.

Sarah begins with an overview:

> For women, it's probably the most emotional side effect. It makes you feel very unattractive. Your self-esteem plummets. . . . It's mad, mad how society reacts. It's just such an awkward situation. People either ignore it because they don't want to bring light to it, or else they stare at you.

She then describes the moment most women who have gone through chemo remember all their lives: She raked her fingers through her hair and found herself clutching a handful of strands.

> I wanted to cry.

She called her brother-in-law and asked him to shave her head. She remembers closing her eyes, waiting for him to finish. When he did,

> I went to my room and cried. I looked in the mirror and it was just too horrible. I just felt horrible.

As the days went by, it bothered her less and less. She put on her makeup and had a realization:

I have a blank canvass to work with.

She realized she could wear pink because it wouldn't clash with her red hair, for example.

It's a crap situation, but you can make the most of it if you want to. . . . It's fun to feel confident in yourself. I think that radiates out. Then (other) people don't mind as much.

Sarah concludes with:

I made this video to give hope to women . . . I'm embracing what I have. The look I have. . . . You can definitely still maintain your beauty. Keep trying. Treat yourself. I know you can do it.[9]

Sarah is admittedly much younger than many gynecologic cancer patients, and she is naturally beautiful. It could be argued, however, that loss of hair would be even worse for someone her age because the "pity factor" associated with a young person with cancer would be considerable. And not being in a long-term relationship yet, she doesn't have a partner to stand shoulder to shoulder with her through this. How much of her newfound confidence would bubble up if she met a person she was sexually attracted to?

But here's the rub: Instead of standing shoulder to shoulder with their cancer-stricken mate, many partners distance themselves. As a corollary, many cancer patients push their partners away instead of inviting them closer for support and love. The numbers from the study are disquieting: 97 percent of the women who reported sexual dysfunction were in long-term relationships. The findings related to the dynamics of a relationship invaded by cancer indicate that the disease and treatment can be as great a threat, or greater, to any relationship as an affair.

- Just 3 percent of the women report that their partner had an affair after the cancer diagnosis. Since many people don't know whether or not their partner has had an affair, this number is probably lower than reality.
- Nearly 15 percent of women who participated in the study engaged in marital counseling with their partner after treatment.
- A little more than 10 percent separated from their partner for a period of time. From an anthropological perspective, any behavior that exceeds a 10 percent rate in a group that is outside of the norm is considered significant.
- Five percent of all women reported divorcing after cancer.

There is some good news also contained in the study. It indicated that certain factors were not significant in these results; namely, length of relationship, if the therapy was surgery and/or radiation alone, where the cancer was located or what stage it was when diagnosed, and race.

One of the most important answers that we gleaned from the study was this: About 35 percent of the survey respondents were in the surveillance phase of their experience. In other words, they were past the cancer. They had already gone through the treatments and were now being monitored to ensure that the disease had not returned.

SOME INSIGHTS FROM THE ANSWERS

We concluded that if 15 percent of the patients are requiring marriage counseling, and some of them are getting divorced as a result of it, the medical community needs to address this reality as part of a holistic approach to cancer care rather than treat cancer simply as a disease.

Let's say you are a Stage I endometrial cancer patient with a 90 to 95 percent chance of being cured. You have your first consult with your doctor, who tells you the good news. You are thrilled! Relieved! Everything is most likely going to be just fine!

And then you learn that, after surgery, your doctor wants to take two additional steps to try to ensure that your type of cancer—even though early stage—is eliminated. He suggests that you have both a short course of chemotherapy and vaginal brachytherapy to take your chances of recurrence as close to zero as possible.

So you have good news that's linked with challenging news about how to make the good news a reality.

But what if he were completely honest with you about the psychosocial ramifications, especially as they pertain to your primary relationship? If the medical community treated your cancer holistically, you would then hear the bleak statistics: You have a 15 percent chance of hitting a rocky shoal in your intimate relationship and separating from your current partner; you have a 100 percent risk of having your sex life be disrupted by the treatment for your disease.

In short, you have about a one in six chance of needing marriage counseling, a one in six chance of separating, and a one in six chance of getting divorced because of your cancer. Now consider this: You are far more likely to have your relationship fall apart than have your cancer come back.

There's another way to look at the percentages, and it's important to go through the exercise. Anyone in the United States, for example, would argue that nearly half of all married couples get divorced. Many of them have gone through some kinds of counseling and chose to split anyway. There are myriad causes; cancer is sometimes one of them. But we're talking about a very specific population in this case: couples affected by gynecologic cancer. There is a source of stress present in the relationship that presents particular challenges to intimacy. It follows, then, that if medical professionals simply managed expectations about how cancer and its treatments can interfere with an intimate relationship, then they might help reduce patients' chances of staying out of the "50 percent pool."

If a doctor is overt about the implications of cancer treatment on sexual functioning, then he or she helps to set expectations. The patient and her partner can prepare for the results to mitigate the negative effects. What's happened most often, though, is that the couple was surprised by the impact: "We didn't expect this!" is what the women would often report.

The little touches and light kisses that were routine suddenly carry a new significance. For a time—maybe weeks and maybe months—that's all you have as a way of displaying your intimate connection to the other person. They mean a lot more and if they aren't given more frequently, both members of the couple can feel isolated and rejected. She feels "alone" because cancer has separated her forcibly from normalcy. Her partner feels "alone" because there is the possibility that he will literally be alone if the treatments don't succeed—alone in the house, alone raising the kids, alone in paying the bills, alone for dinner.

You might be wondering how long this level of attention to detail related to displays of affection needs to persist. As we mentioned above, after the acute phase of the disease and treatment are over, then the couple enters the surveillance, or chronic, phase of the experience. The physical threats are diminished, but the chronic phase is the most treacherous for a relationship. This is actually the period, therefore, when the small expressions of tenderness and flirtatious behavior can become a vital part of the couple's *ongoing* intimacy. And even though the "little things" are important in any relationship, for a couple that has doubts that can linger for years about the survivability of the woman, these signs of caring and desire could be a necessity for the survival of the relationship.

Let's see how this plays out with an ovarian cancer patient whom we would describe as typical.

Ovarian cancer patients tend to first come in when the cancer has reached an advanced stage. Unlike endometrial cancer, for example, there are no very early warning signs that patients easily detect. There may be some bloating or pelvic pain, and perhaps not feeling hungry or urinating a bit more, but these are annoying occurrences that a majority of women would probably attribute to something innocuous unless they persisted.

When ovarian cancer is advanced, it's considered "incurable." It's not that the patient is automatically doomed; the cancer is simply viewed as a chronic issue. The disease may go into remission with the patient never having a recurrence, but technically, a physician would still be reluctant to say the patient is cured.

Here's a common scenario that illustrates the psychological effects of this reality on the patient. She goes through the debulking surgery, which results in a sternum-to-pelvis scar. Then she goes through six rounds of chemotherapy. The CA 125 marker has dropped from 2,000 to 25, so hurrah, she's done with the ordeal for now. Three weeks later, she goes in for her first surveillance visit. She snaps at her husband, is short with the doctor, has nothing warm to say to the nurse, and exhibits other signs of anxiety like fidgeting and rapid breathing.

The doctor asks, "What's wrong?"

"What now?"

"What do you mean, 'what now'?"

She sighs audibly and then lets loose: "It's been four months of treatment and surgery. I have no hair and I have an ugly scar. I'm not 'cured.' I'm just not sick. So what now?"

"Go and enjoy life. There's nothing more to do here. Come and see me every three months and be grateful that your future is just a matter of keeping an eye on things. Bottom line: Stop being a cancer patient."

After diagnosis, the patient knows she needed surgery and chemo, and she plunged into the treatments with diligence. In the surveillance phase, she—and her partner—doesn't feel active. It's like being a soldier who had served in combat being sent to duty at a base eight thousand miles from the battlefield. Still a soldier, but not doing "soldier stuff."

The woman can enter a psychological vortex with the same phrase whipping around and around in her brain: "Will it come back?" The partner may well have the same mental experience—and it's torture for both. Because they aren't doing anything in the same way they were when treatments were in full swing, they can feel even more helpless than they did at the moment of diagnosis. They have seen the enemy and are waiting for it to attack again.

Gynecologic oncologists have reported to us anecdotally that there are ovarian cancer patients in this surveillance phase who check their CA 125 levels every week. They pay private labs to conduct the test because no responsible doctor would order a weekly test and insurance surely wouldn't cover something that is so excessive. If the level "jumps" from 7 to 8, for example, they want to see the doctor. They want a CT scan. They want a battery of tests. It is obsessive behavior that strongly suggests the patient is living in a relationship with cancer rather than with another human being. How would that woman's partner feel?

Knowing what we know from the UC study and others, we have to conclude a couple of overarching things:

1. Most couples should consider going to marriage counseling when they enter the surveillance phase of a cancer, like ovarian, that isn't "curable."
2. Most people who have been treated for cancer should enter some kind of a rehabilitation, or wellness, program to address issues such as neuropathy, fatigue, sleep disturbances, and sexual dysfunction.

In the second half of the book, these and other insights related to the answers we learned from the study will be presented in a prescriptive fashion.

· 4 ·

Like a Rat in a Lab

$\mathscr{F}$or some women, the moment they hear "I'm sorry to tell you this, but you have cancer" is the most devastating moment they have ever known. In terms of inducing stress, however, it can pale in comparison to certain moments during subsequent treatment.

We begin with three events related to treatment that provoke extreme stress for many patients—stress that lingers and is bound to affect sexual functioning for reasons we will explore. We'll also look at studies of stress responses to better understand what behaviors we—and those around us—adopt to mitigate stress in an attempt to return to normal. One is a fascinating piece of work by Robert Sapolsky, the author of *Monkeyluv: And Other Essays on Our Lives as Animals*, who is recognized as one of the country's foremost experts on stress. He shows us that rats in a lab can tell us a great deal about ourselves.

THREE HIGH-STRESS EVENTS

Vaginal Brachytherapy

Amber R. Knuthson is the physician's assistant to Dr. Joshua Petit, a highly regarded radiation oncologist in northern Colorado. She briefs patients on their procedures prior to treatment and is generally the one who remains with the patient during treatment and does the follow-up consults. For that reason, she has a keen perspective on how patients face both their cancer and their treatment. There is one particular type of radiation treatment, however, that gives her insights into the intimate relationships of patients—vaginal brachytherapy.

57

Brachytherapy as a postsurgical, and possibly also a postchemo, treatment for endometrial cancer is done for certain early-stage cases in this practice, so Amber's brachy patients have a high likelihood of survival. You might think that would make them relatively perky and optimistic. That's not necessarily so, and the reason is often related to how the brachy therapy is administered.

In vaginal brachytherapy, a source of radiation is placed into a cylinder and inserted into the vagina. Although the length and girth of the cylinder can vary, the upper part of the vagina is always treated because if there were any "stray" cancer cells remaining after the hysterectomy, this is where they would probably be. The radiation in brachy treatments mainly affects the area of the vagina in contact with the cylinder. Although the bladder and rectum are nearby, they get less radiation exposure.

Vaginal brachy has come a long way in the twenty-first century. Brachytherapy used to mean admission to the hospital and immobility for two to three days while the low-dose radiation was administered on a continuing basis—meaning no going to the bathroom and no getting up and stretching. The source of radiation was inserted in an operating room and then the patient was wheeled on a gurney to her room and placed behind a lead shield. Contrast that with the experience today, with a very targeted, high dose taking a few minutes, and in some cases, fewer than two minutes a session. The downside is that the patient exposed to high-dose treatment is more at risk for long-term side effects like stenosis than someone who has had low-dose treatment.

Amber says that a good many of the vaginal brachy patients she sees have a persistent sense of being violated—first by the cancer, and then by the "invasion" of the radioactive cylinder. Every woman in the Western world probably has an expectation that she will go to a gynecologist once every couple of years and have a pelvic exam. It's invasive, but it doesn't happen very often. As a cancer patient, you go from that to exams that happen monthly or, when you're in the monitoring phase, every three months. And then if you are a vaginal brachy patient, you suddenly have a daily, or every other day, experience for a couple of weeks of having a radioactive cylinder inserted in your body. To exacerbate the feeling of being violated, there is a team of specialists instead of "just" a doctor and nurse monitoring activity in the most private part of your body—the radiation oncologist; a couple of nurses; possibly a physician's assistant and a resident; and a medical physicist, who has helped the doctor plan the treatment and now has a central role in administering it.

The patient knows the experience is for the greater good, so there is going to be some optimism associated with it. Nonetheless, it's hard for even a psychologically and emotionally strong woman to shake the basic, animal feeling that having something foreign repeatedly put in her vagina is a violation of some kind. The sentiment is different from surgery in many ways; most women receive brachytherapy while fully awake, whereas they are asleep and unaware of the examinations during normal surgical procedure.

We want to step back for a moment and note that it's fundamentally no different for a man with prostate cancer. He gets poked and prodded in ways that arouse a sense of violation as well. So whether the patient is male or female, the people around that person need to be aware of how traumatic both the cancer and the treatments can be—and trauma is a stress that can cause odd behaviors, as we will explore later in the chapter.

For some patients, the sense of violation triggers aggression. They are agitated by the cancer and the treatment. For them, the whole experience is like being stuck in a massive traffic jam with nowhere to go and no one telling you when you might start moving again. The dominant emotion is anger, and they sometimes lash out. As we see later in this chapter, that's an effective approach to relieving stress, but it amps up the stress for the person on the receiving end of the anger.

The First Cycle of Chemo

The experience of infusion therapy can engender a sense of violation, too, with the first round offering some jarring surprises to a patient. Although some chemo is given in pill form, we mostly think of it as a therapy administered intravenously, or through the veins. For some patients, they have a new hole in their body to accommodate a port, which is an implanted portal to their circulatory system. For others, chemo means a conventional needle-into-vein delivery system. Both are pathways for medicine to travel from bags hanging from a metal pole through a tube into the body.

When you get checked in at an infusion center, you may see a sunlit room divided into private areas by curtains or other barriers. There are comfortable reclining chairs, beds, chairs for guests, televisions controlled by the patient, and soothing colors. Nurses have smiles and a warm demeanor; they are well aware that you would rather not have to see their smiling faces.

When the treatment is about to begin, one of the nurses who made you comfortable and shared a laugh with you comes toward you wearing a hazmat suit. The formal name is personal protective equipment (PPE), and the nature of it in the United States is determined by the National Institute for Occupational Safety and Health (NIOSH), Occupational Safety and Health Administration (OSHA), American Public Health Association, and the Oncology Nursing Society. Whether your dose is high or low, the nurse wears hair-to-toes covering including double chemotherapy-tested gloves, protective gowns, and protective eyewear if there is a potential for splashing.[1]

That's the moment when patients commonly report an escalating sense of fear, violation, and vulnerability about chemo. They wonder, "What is that stuff in the bag that's dripping into my veins?"

To avert the chances of an allergic reaction, one of the drugs that may be added to the mix is the sedating antihistamine diphenhydramine, or Benadryl®. It takes the edge off the fear and shock by helping you drift toward sleep. But Benadryl eventually wears off.

Removal and Reconstruction of Breasts

We put the two together because we learned how the surgeries for breast cancer are a double whammy of stress, with one not necessarily outweighing the other. One of the patients we interviewed was a young physician whose story illustrates the kind of stress we heard described by so many other breast cancer patients, but hers involved a couple of other pain points that heightened the anxiety: She had both a devastating family history involving this cancer, and she found out about it while she and her husband were undergoing fertility treatments to get pregnant.

A YOUNG DOCTOR'S JOURNEY

Marie's mother passed away of ovarian cancer when Marie was fifteen. Five years before that, she'd gone through breast cancer. So when Marie was in her late twenties, she got tested for the BRCA gene, famously associated with Angelina Jolie, who chose to have preventative breast removal after she tested positive. Marie tested negative, despite the experiences of her mother that would have suggested a genetic predisposition to breast and ovarian cancer. She shelved her concerns.

In her mid-thirties when she went for her first mammogram, Marie immediately got alarming news: "We saw something unusual. You need to go for an MRI." A breast MRI is a relatively new test for high-risk patients that provides super-sensitive imaging to detect abnormalities that a standard mammogram could miss. A powerful magnet is used to take hundreds of images of the breasts both before and after intravenous injection of dye material. The test is much longer than a mammogram, taking about forty-five minutes, and the entire time the patient needs to remain as still as possible to ensure accuracy.

There are mostly advantages to the breast MRI because of its sensitivity. But that level of precision means it can detect both cancerous and benign lesions, and they can appear similar. A patient could be sent off for a biopsy, scared to death, and have nothing more than a benign mass.

Her doctor saw something suspicious and wanted to do the biopsy. Marie was annoyed. She'd had the BRCA test, she felt fine, and she assumed that nothing was wrong. "I was pissed that I had to deal with this," she recalls. Medically speaking, her focus was on fertility treatments so she and her husband Emil could conceive.

Then Marie did something that shows why physicians can make annoying patients. She got the results of her test before her doctor and read them. She saw lobular carcinoma in situ (LCIS) and told Emil. Neither one of them practiced oncology so, having been out of medical school for a while, they had to look up LCIS like any curious layperson. They discovered LCIS was a marker for breast cancer, but not breast cancer. It's an area of abnormal cell growth that would increase Marie's risk of developing invasive breast cancer later. "Lobular" means that the abnormal cells are in the lobules, or milk-producing glands.

Based on the results, she had to have a consultation with a breast surgeon to do more in-depth tests. That first meeting with her new doctor was on her mother's birthday. She needed an open incisional biopsy to take tissue. It's a surgery, done under sedation, but it removes less tissue than an excisional biopsy, which is more commonly known as a lumpectomy.

When Marie went back for her postsurgical consult, the doctor began, "So, I have to talk to you . . ." Not a good beginning. She continued, "We sent your pathology report out for a second opinion and they read your pathology as DCIS." That's good news wrapped in bad news for a patient with breast cancer. Ductal carcinoma in situ (DCIS) is the most common type of noninvasive breast cancer. According to BreastCancer.org, "Ductal means that the cancer starts inside the milk ducts, carcinoma refers to any cancer that begins in the skin or other tissues (including breast tissue) that cover or line the internal organs, and in situ means 'in its original place.'"[2] It's noninvasive because it hasn't spread beyond the milk duct into the surrounding breast tissue, but the presence of it puts you at high risk for cancer coming back. With DCIS, the odds of a recurrence are about one in three.

Marie made an intense effort to learn about her options—not from Internet searches but by interviewing people within and outside of the medical community who had direct experience with a DCIS diagnosis. Her advantage was being a physician, as well as being married to a physician on staff at a major medical center. She concluded that she would follow the advice of the people who really know what they were talking about—including her fertility doctor: have a bilateral mastectomy.

Marie found herself in a state of shock after enduring a five-hour surgery to remove the tissue from both breasts and implant tissue expanders:

> In my head, I'd minimized the surgery. I convinced myself it wasn't going to be a big deal. And it was horrible. It was so much worse than I thought it would be. And the recovery was horrible. I couldn't take any pain medication. The narcotics made me dizzy or nauseated or constipated or agitated. And I wasn't allowed to take ibuprofen because it affects bleeding.
>
> The worst pain was two weeks. It was like being stabbed in the chest over and over. I went back to work at four weeks and it was really hard. If I moved the wrong way, it felt like I was tearing apart. I would wake up crying at night.

In our interview, we also asked Emil how *he* felt about his beautiful wife's double mastectomy:

> I felt really sad, but in my mind it was not a question of what to do; it was a matter of doing it. I think being in medicine gave me a really good perspective on it. I'd treated a lot of patients with cancer in my residency and they taught me to be an optimist. The fact that Marie would not need radiation therapy or chemotherapy was, to me, a blessing.
>
> Many times in our relationship, Marie tends to be the pessimist and I tend to be the optimist. This was one of those times the difference was evident! My attitude was, "Let's get this done."
>
> For me, the most scary part was after the biopsy. Seeing my own wife in a hospital gown after years of seeing patients in hospital gowns—that was horrible.
>
> But I think the most heartbreaking time of the whole event—she may not even remember this—is we stayed in the hospital one night after her surgery. They wheeled her into the room about six o'clock. She was taking pain medicine. One of the doctors came by at about nine or ten to look at the wounds. Protocol. And when Marie said, "I can't look! I can't look!" that's when I broke down. I had built up a wall, thinking, "We'll cut this cancer out and move on with our life." It was hard seeing her in so much pain—pain of all kinds.

Marie had been a side sleeper, so having to sleep on her back for weeks added to her discomfort. In fact, Emil says she woke up almost every night crying in pain—sometimes screaming in pain. The narcotics made her vomit, so she had a choice between acute pain and acute nausea. According to the patients we interviewed, that's a common story. She also couldn't lift her arms, so her husband and mother-in-law had to cook, help her dress, bathe her, and even brush her hair.

For the two weeks after the surgery, she also needed help with the drains coming out of her sides. This is plastic tubing coming out of the side of the rib cage, hanging out a few inches below the armpit. These tubes drain the breast for any blood that might be pooling; it pours into a bulb that must be emptied every few hours.

As a successful physician with her own practice—a take-charge individual—Marie found the challenge of dependency on others more stressful than the surgery itself because it lingered. She found herself snapping at the very people who helped her most, almost as though it were somehow their fault that she couldn't help herself. And when remorse over her behavior would set in, then she would berate herself and turn inward. She discovered what psychologists and psychiatrists have been trying to tell our stressed-out society for years: Chronic stressful life situations can be a huge risk factor for depression.

Physical therapy helped Marie regain her range of motion. She was also regaining some strength. She needed it because the next hurdle, which she thought would be "no big deal" compared to the mastectomy, was higher than the last one in terms of pain and inconvenience. It was time to get new breasts.

Her reconstructive surgery involved expanding the balloons that had been implanted to stretch the surrounding tissues and skin and then a surgery to give her the permanent implants. The balloons were filled with an increasing amount of saline to gently expand the region to make room for the implants chosen by the patient. If you want to be a D cup ultimately, you need a lot more saline than the patient who's happy as a B. The expanders are hard, too—like having a couple of rocks in your chest.

This is not without humor. Marie had been a D cup who chose to go to a B. Emil reminded her that this would eliminate any career changes that would take her to Las Vegas.

Three months later, Marie went back into surgery to get her implants. Since this is surgery that many women choose for cosmetic purposes, it has a reputation of being a much less stressful experience than a mastectomy. According to the American Society of Plastic Surgeons (ASPS), breast augmentation surgery is the top-ranked cosmetic surgical procedure in the United States. The 2015 number hit nearly three hundred thousand.

But Marie didn't start the journey with an eye on looking sexier. She was pushed down this road and couldn't shake the association between breast surgery and cancer. Facing the implantation surgery was, of course, a hopeful time, but in her mind it still carried the stigma of "cancer therapy."

Even though she was warned not to draw any conclusions about the cosmetic results for six months, she found herself constantly looking at herself in the mirror. She thought they looked asymmetrical, or weird, or lumpy, depending on the day. She hammered her self-esteem with negative adjectives, despite the fact that her husband deemed them "perfect."

Not touching for many weeks was perhaps the hardest part of the experience. They still wanted to have a baby, but physically, it was uncomfortable to be close. And the stress of feeling damaged and ugly—going from a striking brunette with a shapely body to a pain-ridden, surgically altered cancer patient—put Marie's desire on the ice. The realization that sensations in the breast area were not returning was another reminder that their intimacy wouldn't be the same.

> After all that, I was afraid to have him touch me. I didn't want anything to happen to them. I was worried they would rupture and then I'd have to have *more* surgery. The thought of bumping into something hard or falling on a sidewalk would freak me out.
>
> I went back to exercising after six weeks and every time I moved an arm and felt something, I thought I'd torn something. I was fearful so much of the time.

In her head and her heart, Marie knew her husband would love her no matter what. And yet that pair of aesthetic attributes that had first attracted him to her was gone. In its place was a pair that would frequently remind them both that she'd had cancer. They needed time to move forward and, in the meantime, Marie says that daily life "was very, very stressful."

When they had sexual intercourse after the surgeries were completed, Emil said the experiences were a little off-putting at first. He touched her breast erotically and she felt nothing. She also had concern that his touching her breast would "explode the implants." So they had to work around the new additions for a while.

As the interviews for this book were nearly completed, we spoke again with Emil who said they were both breathing easier now that they had had a full six months postreconstruction to heal and recharge. And, he said with great happiness, "We are pregnant."

STRESS AND SEXUAL DYSFUNCTION

Regardless of what kind of patient you are, if you're being treated for cancer you have more stress than usual in your life. Usually, it's related to a convergence of factors that might include fear of the disease, missing work, concern over appearance, and insufficient financial resources. Your partner is probably experiencing stress, probably for some of the same reasons. Regardless of what you are capable of doing physically, the stress will pay a role in your sex life, even to the point where stress alone completely derails it.

Robert Sapolsky, PhD is a professor of biological sciences and a professor of neurology and neurological sciences at Stanford University. He explains the concept of stress as follows:

> Homeostasis is having an ideal body temperature, an ideal level of glucose in the bloodstream, an ideal everything. That's being in homeostatic balance.
>
> A stressor is anything in the outside world that knocks you out of homeostatic balance. . . . So to reestablish that balance, you secrete adrenaline and other hormones. You mobilize energy and you deliver it where it's needed, you shut off the inessentials like the sex drive and digestion, you enhance immune defenses, and you think more clearly. You're facing a short-term physical crisis, and the stress response is what you do with your body. For 99 percent of the species on this planet, stress is three minutes of screaming terror in the savannah, after which either it's over with or you're over with. That's all you need to know about the subject if you're a zebra or a lion.
>
> If you're a human, though, you've got to expand the definition of a stressor in a very critical way. If you're running from a lion, your blood pressure is 180 over 120. But you're not suffering from high blood pressure—you're saving your life. Have this same thing happen when you're stuck in traffic, and you're not saving your life. Instead you are suffering from stress-induced hypertension.[3]

Sapolsky offers a brief explanation of "Why Stress Creates Erectile Dysfunction" to give us all the data points we need to understand how stress gets in the way of sex. The background necessary for this is a basic understanding of the parasympathetic and sympathetic nervous systems. The parasympathetic is all about calm, about feeling secure and comforted. The sympathetic is notably associated with emergency action, as in a state of fight or flight. All systems are "go," as he described in the above paragraphs. Keep in mind that this description is about men, but the essential message is true for women as well:

> In order to get an erection, you've got to turn on the parasympathetic nervous system. You've got to be calm and vegetative. Okay, so you got your erection. What happens next? Maybe something to do with the social context that brought about the erection in the first place—maybe you start feeling a little less calm and vegetative. Maybe you start breathing a little bit faster. Maybe your heart rate increases. Maybe you're beginning to expend some muscular energy. Maybe you're beginning to turn on the sympathetic nervous system. And more time goes by and you're breathing faster, and your heart's racing, and eventually your toes are curling, and

you're sweating, and you're turning on the sympathetic nervous system throughout the whole body, except there's one lone outburst where you're desperately holding on to the parasympathetic as long as possible. Finally, you can't take it anymore and you turn off the parasympathetic and turn on the sympathetic and you ejaculate.[4]

He concludes this talk by noting how devastating the presence of stress is to healthy sexual functioning. Sapolsky says that 60 percent of the doctor visits in the United States for erectile dysfunction don't result from any organic problem, but rather the problem relates to stress.

WHAT THE RATS TELL US

In a study of how rats handled stress, Sapolsky set up scenarios involving different options for rats to alleviate the pain that very tense situations imposed on them. He put two cages side by side, with a rat in each case. Each rat would get a shock that mimicked what happened to the other, so it would be the same intensity, duration, and moment in time. The difference is that only one of the rats gets the shock, whereas the other is subjected to a bit of psychological manipulation.

Here is how the rats that had options to alleviate stress behaved:

- In one case, after the rat got shocked he could run across the case to where another rat was—one that didn't get shocked—and bite him. The "victim" rat served as an outlet for the other rat's anger. In human terms, you share the stress with someone else by picking on him. Whether you're a rat or a person, this can be effective in dramatically reducing stress, but it is abusive.
- When Marie was telling her story, she admitted that she would occasionally lash out the people who helped her. Even though that sounds ungrateful and rude, it's normal. The shocked rat that takes out his frustration and anger by biting the other rat isn't a deranged killer, he's sharing the pain.

Sapolsky explains the dynamic and helps set the stage for some of the antistress guidance that shows up in part II:

It's documented by science. It [taking it out on someone else] makes you feel better, which is why the first sound bite they have you do in stress management is "Don't reduce your chance of getting an ulcer by giving it to somebody else. Make sure your outlets are not abusive ones."[5]

In the next scenario, after the rat gets shocked, he can go over to the other side of the case and gnaw on wood. He still gets an outlet, but he isn't hurting another rat. In human terms, this means dissipating the stress through a hobby, exercise, project at work, or maybe by making elaborate lunches for your elementary school children. The activity is an outlet that does the job of relieving tension and frustration, but it isn't abusive.

- This approach can cut two ways. It is a better way to go than yelling at your caregiver—and if you're exercising, for example, it could lead to great health benefits—but it can also indicate an avoidance of your reality.
- Barbara threw herself into volunteer work at her local hospital after she learned she had ovarian cancer. Her doctor and treatments were both located at the same hospital so she had a fever for helping others with cancer. But unlike most people at the hospital, she had tremendous financial means so she could pay bills for state-of-the-art treatment. All she knew was that she didn't want any woman to be denied the level of treatment she had because they didn't have the money or the insurance to cover the costs. The gala she orchestrated raised more than a million dollars for women who needed financial help. She felt great! But she also wore herself out and suffered a setback with her own healing. Her doctor said, "Barbara, you will have years to help other people if you take care of yourself now."

The third situation in Sapolsky's experiment gave the rat a warning. Ten seconds before he would receive a shock, a light went on. It's true for humans as well as rats: Add a degree of predictability to the stressful experience and you're much better off. When the mind knows when a stressful event is coming and has a sense of how bad it will be, then the reaction to it is less severe.

- Every cancer patient gets used to the blood draw. It's a routine part of keeping tabs on your medical profile. Even if you've done this a dozen times before, though, it's essentially unpleasant. The medical technician will probably say every time, "You'll feel a little sting when I put the needle in, but it will go away quickly." The technician's words add a bit of additional predictability that the patient appreciates. Similarly, the experience of vaginal brachytherapy at a facility like Joshua Petit's, where the equipment allows the medical physicist to stay in the room with the patient during treatment, involves a countdown. The patient knows there are sixty seconds remaining, twenty seconds, and then the happy words, "All done!" Even though there is no pain whatsoever involved in the treatment, for reasons cited above, there is still stress for most patients.

- Lynne was one of the patients who contributed to the study, and she added a story that shows the powerful value of predictability. Her dear friend Penny had gone through the diagnosis and treatment of endometrial cancer just six months prior to her own diagnosis. Penny was the first person that Lynne called when her doctor gave her the unsettling news. Penny told her, "It's a straightforward surgery. You'll be in the hospital just a night or two. . . ." As she listened to Penny describe what was ahead, Lynne could feel her heart rate and breathing return to normal. It was as though she had been in a dark room, afraid of the dark, and then Penny opened a door and flicked the light switch.

In the final scenario, the rat feels he has a degree of control over the possibility of a stressful event. He learns that if he presses a lever, there is a chance he will decrease the likelihood of a shock. Sometimes it works and sometimes it doesn't, but the fact that it works sometimes makes him try to exercise control by pounding that lever. Similarly, for the patient who has a sense of control and decision making related to the stressful experience of cancer treatment, that feeling minimizes the stress response. "Control makes stressors less stressful," according to Sapolsky.[6]

- Although health care professionals are trained to ask questions that yield some control to the patient—"Is there a pain medication you prefer?"—the patient's partner, family, and friends may take actions that wrest control from the patient. In an effort to be "helpful," they might present a tray of food without asking, "Are you hungry?" or "What would you like to eat?" They might suggest, "Let's try to go the bathroom now" when all she wants to do is sleep. All of those little control-stealing actions can make the stress of recovery worse. Not only does the patient feel physically weak from treatment but also she feels psychologically weak because she isn't "allowed" to make any basic decisions for herself. It's demoralizing.
- A number of questions in the UC study approach the issue of the patient's sense of control in the context of the intimate relationship. Consider how stressful it would be for a patient who has people around her undercutting her decision about what to eat and when to go to the bathroom when she also would say "true" to these descriptions of her partner's behavior:

Wants me to take his/her side in an argument
Wants to know exactly what I'm doing and where I am

Is clearly hurt if I don't accept his/her views
Tends to try and change me
Seeks to dominate me
Tends to control everything I do

It's easy to envision a woman with a cancer diagnosis as being one of Sapolsky's lab rats. Four scenarios linked to four ways of managing stress. What is probably true for most patients is that each of the scenarios seems familiar, reflecting behaviors and options at different points in time. There is no Dr. Sapolsky orchestrating these scenarios, but it could be argued that a patient's medical team and partner can play a Sapolsky-like role in the patient's stress responses.

Let's focus on the predictability and control scenarios for a moment here, and then return to them in part II. A patient with a healthy amount of intellectual curiosity can have the cancer experience be part of an awakening—about the specifics of her treatment, about her potential to heal and thrive, and about her relationships. The patient's medical team and partner, particularly, have opportunities to make her feel like Alice in Wonderland.

> "Curiouser and curiouser!" cried Alice (she was so much surprised, that for the moment she quite forgot how to speak good English); "now I'm opening out like the largest telescope that ever was! Good-bye, feet!" (for when she looked down at her feet, they seemed to be almost out of sight, they were getting so far off). "Oh, my poor little feet, I wonder who will put on your shoes and stockings for you now, dears? I'm sure *I* shan't be able! I shall be a great deal too far off to trouble myself about you: you must manage the best way you can—but I must be kind to them," thought Alice, "or perhaps they won't walk the way I want to go! Let me see: I'll give them a new pair of boots every Christmas."
>
> —Lewis Carroll, *Alice's Adventures in Wonderland*

Although Lewis Carroll is describing the strange condition of Alice growing to the stature of a giant after eating morsels of an enchanted cake, there are patients who come to have a similar reaction to many aspects of the cancer experience. They are surprised and frightened, of course, but with the help of their medical team and partner, an irresistible curiosity about the entire process keeps them wondering "what's next?" They rely on the predictability of certain experiences and appreciate the degree to which they are in control of their lives.

The woman's body is suddenly strange to her after a cancer diagnosis. Things are happening; things are being done to her to effect inexplicable changes. Yet if people around her answer her questions, they support her sense of control and drive her curiosity, then concurrently they reduce her stress. She gets answers to "what" and "why" and makes choices that affect "what next."

This is the path away from stress and toward homeostasis.

The New Normal

There is a significant decline in a woman's sexual function after undergoing treatment for gynecological cancers. This decline in sexual function can have a detrimental effect on a survivor's quality of life and marital relationships.

—Saketh Guntupalli, author of sexual health study

I was always a thong wearer before. I had a cute little body to go into my cute little underwear. Now he would see my granny pants.

—Allis, a survey participant who had a pelvic exenteration

In addition to the sexual dysfunction research covered in previous chapters, a study led by physicians at Massachusetts General Hospital in Boston found that up to 70 percent of women with cancer reported significant sexual dysfunction. For the most part, they had resigned themselves to thinking there was "nothing that could be done." Other dire results, backed up by statistics, indicate that a lot of women seem to give up when they face sexual and marital dysfunction after cancer.

And then, what we have found in our gynecologic oncology practice is that there are women who come along and have lessons for everyone about keeping sex and love alive. They rethink their love lives, they and their partners adjust, and they discover new paths to satisfaction in their relationship.

In the following story, which is the centerpiece of this presentation on the "new normal," we intersperse essential explanatory information about testing, patient-doctor interaction, therapies, emotional responses, cognitive dissonance, and even spirituality throughout the story. These elements are all integral to the story; they are necessary to illuminate facts, lessons, and insights that are important to this patient and her husband and their message to other women and their partners. We also need to point out that the quotes are the recollections of the patient and her husband; they are spoken words as they remember them with no recorders involved in the original conversations. Finally, the patient's name and selected other details have been altered to protect the identity of her, her husband, and their children.

And now, we introduce you to Allis and Craig.

THE ROUGH ROAD TO "NEW NORMAL"

If it's possible to have a routine day in a third-grade classroom, Allis was having one. She lugged around a few science projects and set them up in the classroom. A tank of guppies, a big plastic model of an ear—she placed them on desks and got the students talking about each one. At the end of the day, she realized her back hurt. She mentioned it to a fellow teacher who was also a massage therapist who said, "Go to your primary care physician first and have him write a prescription for massage therapy so we can run it through your insurance."

A few days later, with the backache getting really annoying by the end of the school day, Allis had her appointment with the doctor. She asked for a prescription for massages.

"Nope," he replied. "I believe in massages only for fun. If you have a backache, you're going to mask a symptom with massages." He said he thought she might have fibroids and ordered an ultrasound.

His suspicion was logical. Although a lot of women who have them don't have any symptoms, some women experience heavy menstrual bleeding, prolonged periods, pelvic pain, problems with urination, constipation, and/or backaches. Saying "maybe you have fibroids" wasn't a scary speculation, and it did start the process of critical testing.

Allis recalls that her ultrasound was a little upsetting: "I noticed the technician stayed on the right side a looooong time."

Right afterward, she got a phone call from her doctor's nurse. She told her, "The doctor wants you to do one more blood test."

"What? I've already had a battery of blood tests."

"He wants you to have a CA 125 test." CA 125 stands for "cancer antigen 125." It's a protein that may reach elevated levels in the blood of patients with certain types of cancers. The test that Allis's doctor ordered is used to help detect early signs of ovarian cancer. It is *not* a 100 percent accurate way of determining if a woman has ovarian cancer because noncancerous conditions can also cause elevation of the CA 125 levels. In fact, even the presence of fibroids can cause an increased level of CA 125. At the same time, it's a tool that helps a physician move up the decision tree toward a diagnosis.

Allis had no idea what CA 125 was. "It sounds like a sports car, so I guess this could be fun," she joked. Silence. "So what is it?"

"It's not something I can discuss with you. I'll ask the doctor to call you."

At this point in the story, we're going to interject some advice for doctors. When Maryann's test results came back as questionable, the first person to call her was the physician himself. Even though that causes heart thumps and sweating, it was reassuring in the sense that he was the source of answers and thoughts on next steps. Having a nurse or other assistant call and not be allowed to answer basic questions is a lapse in patient care.

Not getting an answer from the nurse, Allis did a Google search on the term *CA 125*. She found lots of entries like this one from MedicineNet:

CA 125 is a protein that is a so-called tumor marker or biomarker, which is a substance that is found in greater concentration in tumor cells than in other cells of the body. In particular, CA 125 is present in greater concentration in ovarian cancer cells than in other cells. It was first identified in the early 1980s, and the function of the CA 125 protein is not currently understood.[1]

To say that this frightened Allis is an understatement. She felt the blood rush through her body in a typical "fight-flight-or-freeze" response. The sympathetic nervous system immediately wakes up when the body senses a threat. Stress hormones flood the body; the impulse is to punch, run, or sit paralyzed in the hope that nothing will harm you.

The next call Allis received was from her doctor's office saying, "The doctor wants to see you."

"Okay, I'll make an appointment."

"Today. Can you come after school?" And then Allis learned that her CA 125 level shouldn't be any higher than 35 and it was 200. As a "by the way," she learned there was a chance she could have ovarian cancer and it would be wise to make an appointment with her gynecologist.

At the time, Allis lived in a small, rural town. She had never even heard of a gynecologic oncologist (aka "gyn onc"), so she went to her gynecologist.

In telling her story, Allis laughed in the kind of reflective, how-could-I-be-so-blind way that a smart woman laughs in talking about bad decisions. She said her gynecologist said, "Yep. Elevated CA 125 levels. I'll do a complete hysterectomy." Not getting any verbal response from her—she was again experiencing the fight-flight-or-freeze reaction caused by her sympathetic nervous system—he added, "I'm used to doing this. No problem. When I get in there, if there's anything unusual, I can scrape it, and if there's anything of concern, I'll send it off for a biopsy."

Allis greenlighted the surgery. This was in 2010, and she and Craig both admit to being very naïve about what they faced. They had never had any major health issues, and they made an assumption that "surgery and a little chemo would take care of it and we'd go on with our life," as Craig recalls. "Originally, we didn't really understand the disease and grasp that it was not curable."

In retrospect, she learned that the best decision would have been to go to a gynecologic oncologist rather than a gynecologist. Her gynecologist even articulated his speculation to her and her husband that he was "pretty sure" her problem wasn't cancer. After he did the procedure, it was a very different story.

> My mom, my dad, and my husband sat in the waiting room of the hospital during my surgery. They told me that my gynecologist walked into the room with his head hanging and said, "I'm sorry. Well, we were wrong." He had found all kinds of problems.

Three days later, she got a call that she needed a bowel resection because the surgeon had taken a scrape off her bowel and found it was cancerous. So days after she had gone home to recuperate from the hysterectomy, Allis went back to the hospital to have a piece of her bowel removed.

Soon after that, Allis and her husband found an oncologist in the area. But he was a general oncologist. It's important to note here that physicians who address a broad range of diseases and injuries are vital to the integrity of the medical system. And then, depending on where on the continuum of issues—from common to unique—that a patient lies, the role of a subspecialist becomes less or more important.

The oncologist within a reasonable driving distance of her rural community got her into a trial treatment program that involved her having two ports for chemotherapy: chest and abdomen.

Have you ever seen someone you know is in cancer treatment who has a "lump" about half an inch high on his shoulder area or head, for example? This is an implanted port. The port is like an artificial vein—a bigger-than-normal vein—and it allows medicine to be delivered to the bloodstream efficiently. Ports generally stay implanted for years and make repeated treatments and blood draws more comfortable for the patient than being stuck in the arm, or somewhere else, time after time. Implanted ports should never hurt. A port is a two-part system, with the port serving as a container for fluids that are injected. The lower part is the catheter, which is a small, flexible tube that sits under the skin and connects with a large vein that goes to the heart. A special needle is used to put medication into the port or draw fluids out of it.

The chemotherapy that Allis received in the two ports was different. She describes the abdominal chemo as "medicine being swished around my insides." She recalls having to get on her hands and knees during the infusion and putting her head near the floor. For those readers familiar with yoga, it would be like the *marjariasana*, or cat tilt pose.

She then received Avastin, the trade name for bevacizumab, which is the first clinically used angiogenesis inhibitor. In other words, it's a substance designed to slow the growth of new blood vessels. Avastin works by interfering with the formation of blood vessels that feed the tumor, and the Food and Drug Administration approved it in 2004 for use with chemotherapy for a limited number of cancers. One of them was ovarian. Allis went in to have Avastin administered through her chest port every week for several weeks.

The doctor then told her she was cancer-free.

Five months and three weeks later, Allis got a backache. "It was the exact same backache I'd had before, and I kept telling my husband, 'No, I'm scared.' He said, 'No! They said you're cancer-free!'"

Allis went to her oncologist who ordered at CT scan ("computerized tomography"), which is a useful image in determining the stage of a cancer. He also ordered an MRI and a PET scan. The MRI (magnetic resonance imaging) is useful in distinguishing between normal and diseased tissue. The PET (positron emission tomography), like the CT scan, helps reveal the presence and severity of a cancer.

Allis learned that her cancer was back—aggressively back.

Allis and Craig went to a big city nearby to a gynecologic oncologist who scolded her: "You should have had your first surgery done with me." She took a breath, not being in the mood to be scolded. They recall that the doctor continued, "You could have avoided a lot if you had seen a gyn onc in the first place."

It's possible that Allis and Craig have a flawed recollection of the doctor's tone of voice and attitude. After all, they were both in an emotional state and maybe to them it sounded as though the doctor was scolding. Then again, the doctor's message, regardless of the actual tone of voice, is a berating one. Instead of simply getting on with the consultation and outlining the next steps, the doctor took the time to diminish the decisions they had made before. From a psychological perspective, this is rocky beginning with the doctor. It foreshadowed a rocky end as well.

The gyn onc explained that she would do an exploratory surgery. She said that, when she got in there, she would do whatever she needed to do to get Allis back into her cancer-free state.

During the surgery, the gyn onc rerouted one of Allis's ureters, which is a duct that passes urine. She also took a tumor out of Allis's bladder, and then said, "Good to go." With another few sessions of chemo, Allis thought the threat was behind her.

Allis is a petite and beautiful woman. She lost her hair during the first round of chemo; it grew back. Then she lost it again during the second round that featured Gemzar (gemcitabine), which was approved by the Food and Drug Administration in 2006 and is used as part of the therapy to treat ovarian cancer patients who have relapsed.[2]

Three months after she completed the chemo, Allis got a backache.

The CT scan indicated that the cancer was back on her ureter. The gyn onc who had been treating her, and had done the resection on her ureter previously, called her regular gynecologist—not Allis—and declared that this case was beyond her abilities and this was the end of the road. She was done.

Allis phoned her office repeatedly and never got a return call. All she wanted to do was say, "*I'm* not done!" Her gynecologist then counseled her on all the treatments that, supposedly, could no longer be used to help her. The message was: "Get your affairs in order."

Throughout the grueling chemo, the loss of hair, the severity of the surgeries, and the emotional trauma, Craig displayed his love for Allis in little and big ways. The first time Allis was losing her hair, he found a hair stylist who had done a lot of work with cancer patients and hired her to come to the house. She shaved off Allis's long blond hair, and then gave them insights on how the hair might grow back, when to expect it to look normal, and what kind of wigs and scarves she might consider. It's one of the many tough things they did together, although he did lighten the mood when he reminded Allis that he just couldn't relate to her trauma because he was already bald. The next day, he gave Allis a dozen roses—the first of many dozens, since he still surprises her with flowers.

Just after Allis got the news that her gyn onc was done with her, there was a turn of events that seemed destined to exacerbate the emotional and physical stress that the couple was going through: Craig was transferred to a city a thousand miles away. He set up a commuting schedule until Allis could find someone to take her classroom.

So after she got the news that she had very little time to live, she drove home in the rain to an empty house and cried. Her aunt arrived soon after, but their hugs and tears were interrupted. They heard what sounded like a waterfall. The gutters had overflowed.

Allis and her aunt headed outside, and Allis climbed up a ladder to pull leaves out of the gutter.

> It's pouring rain. My aunt is down on the ground holding a bucket. I'm grabbing leaves out of the gutter and crying, "I'm not done! I'm just not ready to be done! This just sucks!" By the time we finished clearing the gutters, we were plastered in leaves and mud and we laughed so hard. We laughed and laughed and then she said, "You know, the only thing we can do right now is to pray." So we did.

At the end of December, Allis moved to where her husband had been transferred—Denver, Colorado. She arrived in her new cancer clinic distraught and scared. Once again, she heard that the prognosis wasn't good. She probably had a few months left and additional surgery wasn't advisable. Craig recalls: "We pushed Dr. Guntupalli for a number. Three months? Four months? We want to know how to prepare. We want to be ready."

But Allis took a giant step past that and told her new doctor, "A few months is not acceptable." She gave him a kind of ultimatum: "Keep me alive at least until my son graduates from high school. I need you to help me get there." That meant that Allis was "demanding" at least another three years of life. She saw a glimmer of hope in the response: "We will do everything in our power to make that possible. With two recurrences, the odds that you'll make it another three years are slim—but they aren't zero."

Allis had a tumor growing on her rectum that showed accelerated growth, so even though surgery was not advisable, "advisable" was out the window. She would have to have surgery or the tumor would perforate her bowel. Strangely, though, this was the only site of cancer that she had; the rest of her abdomen appeared to be free of cancer. Craig framed the procedure as a way to control his wife's death rather than have it be an emergency. The surgery wouldn't cure her—not by a long shot—but it might allow them more time together to plan a death with dignity. They could go through the items on their mutual bucket list and try to enjoy their remaining time together.

Keep in mind that he had to sustain his career throughout these multiple ordeals so that their family health insurance would remain current and they had some kind of income. He needed twice as much energy, he needed to survive on far less sleep than most people, just to make life work for them on a day-to-day basis. And with the bucket list, they also had committed to having time for fun together.

The scheduled surgery—the surgery Craig saw as "an attempt to keep her death under control"—was estimated to take six hours. Craig and his parents camped in the waiting area, prepared to be there the whole day. Craig had his laptop so he could work remotely rather than claim vacation time or sick leave. After just two hours, a nurse came out and approached Craig with "The doctor would like to see you."

His heart broke. He jumped to the conclusion that they had lost Allis on the table.

Craig froze as Allis's surgeon walked across the waiting room toward him. Craig recalls:

> The blood had drained out of my face. I felt limp and numb. He sounded committed and focused as he told me they found the tumor they were looking for, but while they were looking around, there were other tumors

visible—like five on the bladder, rectum, colon, one going down the artery on her leg—and just about everywhere. But he said they thought they could get the cancer. All of it.

What he proposed is a surgery "of last resort" called a total pelvic exenteration. This radical procedure removes all the organs from the pelvic cavity, and for a woman that means removal not only of the urinary bladder, urethra, rectum, and anus but also the female organs. Since Allis had already had surgery to remove her uterus, she was looking at removal of her vagina and cervix. The surgery results in a permanent colostomy and urinary diversion, so the person must wear two small bags to collect urine and feces.

Craig faced a decision: Stick with an estimated three more months of life for his wife, or go for the possibility of years with this radical surgery. "What would Allis want?" he asked himself. The answer was, "Years."

After eleven and a half hours of surgery, Allis woke up to good news and bad news. The good news was that her prognosis was much better than before the surgery; it appeared that all signs of cancer had been removed. The bad news, which paled in comparison, was that she would have two little bags attached to her abdomen for the rest of her life. But at least it now seemed possible that she would have a life.

Craig's first thought was, "I have to be the rock, the one to lift her when she's down. I've got to be one-through-ten—everything she needs all the time. And I want to keep the romance alive." It was a noble set of goals, but cancer and its aftermath challenge even the clearest intentions and best-laid plans.

When Allis and Craig got married, they had a pact to always keep their romance alive, and they had developed special rituals and habits that supported that intent. One of them was, as Allis says, "We would never toot in front of each other. We would go into another room." While she was still in the hospital and acclimating to her colostomy, Allis realized, "It toots. It talks."

> The first time it happened—with Craig in the room—I threw my hands up in the air and went, "Aaaack!"
> Craig said, "What?!"
> "Did you hear that? I farted! It was really long!" I was devastated.
> "I didn't hear it. If you hadn't screamed and thrown your arms in the air, I wouldn't have known."

This was the beginning of a "new normal" for Allis and Craig. The subsequent chemo and radiation was followed by yet another cancer scare.

This time, an intensive series of radiation treatments—every workday for a month—beat the disease.

But (we know you don't want to see this word in this story any more, do you?) Allis then developed fistulas. A fistula is a hole—an abnormal connection between two hollow spaces. At this point, she had faith in her medical team, her husband, and her God that the problem would be mitigated after treatment, but she was screaming in pain. The fistulas meant that digestive fluid was leaking into parts of her body not designed to deal with acid.

Allis had already established the "Ritual of 24 Hours." Ever since her first cancer diagnosis, she had asked everyone around her to give her twenty-four hours to be nuts. She knew that crying, acting irrationally, and punching a stuffed animal might alleviate her stress. It did help, and so she repeated it all those times that someone called and put her into fight-flight-or-freeze mode again.

This time, though, the leaking acid caused blistering and intense pain. Crying was not an option to release anxiety; it was the only response she had to her suffering.

Her after-hours call of desperation quickly reached her doctor, who happened to be in Australia. "I can't stand this pain," she said. He flew back to perform surgery—surgery that the entire team knew would be stressful for her body, but there was no choice.

Groggy, but still slightly conscious, Allis remembers being in the surgical suite and hearing the words, "Has everybody eaten?" The question was repeated, followed by the order, "I don't want anyone passing out." That suggested that the surgery might be long and demanding.

Allis woke up with no pain, relatively speaking. With mesh inside her that blocks the abnormal openings, she was able to resume the "new normal" that she and Craig had embarked on.

After all she had gone through, Allis reflected on something she had discussed with her doctor's nurse when she had lived in a place one thousand miles away from her current home. When tumors had invaded one part of her pelvic region, and then another, the subject of total pelvic exenteration had entered their conversation. The nurse whispered, "Oh, honey, you don't want a urostomy. You'll be the stinky one in the room." Allis confronted her doctor. Would you ever do it, she wondered? "Absolutely not. You don't ever want to do something like that. The quality of your life will be horrible. You won't want to live."

How wrong she was.

Now we come to the second phase of Allis's story: the real dive into what constitutes a "new normal" in terms of quality-of-life activities, including sexual intimacy.

ENJOYING THE "NEW NORMAL"

Before delving into the specifics of how Allis and Craig restored their love life, it's important to note how Allis and other cancer survivors felt that the people around them made *practical* contributions to their ultimate health and well-being. Those we interviewed emphasized the roles of many different people from many different circles.

> I feel great. I did Jodi's walk this year. [Jodi's Race for Awareness is a 5K and one-mile run/walk in Denver, Colorado.] I walked with a Stage III B two-year cancer survivor. It's amazing the people I met there—and the stories. Everyone has a story . . . and we are not willing to give up. We thank our doctors, and we thank our God.

> We went back to the church we used to attend when we lived in our other home and the pastor saw us and acknowledged me in front of the whole congregation with: "How many of you have ever seen a walking miracle? We have one in our church today. Someone we have said many prayers for, day after day."

At this point in the interview, which took place in Allis's home, Maryann happened to mention that her own experience of healing began days before her surgery and subsequent chemo and radiation with a Mass that included very close friends. She added that one of those friends then presented her with a prayer shawl, knitted by women from the church who "infused the shawl with prayer and love." Before she could even finish her sentence, Allis jumped up and down and then grabbed Maryann's hand, racing with her into an adjoining room: draped on a chair was Allis's prayer shawl.

For nonbelievers or believers, the point of this is something Allis summarized as follows: "When it really matters, people are so generous in giving whatever tangible and intangible gifts they have to offer to help you."

Craig gave both kinds of gifts daily. The two of them never lost hope that they would find a way to restore their love life. But the journey was not without a few surprises.

> We gave it about six months before we tried having sex. Part of the reason for waiting was to be sure I was healed and part of it was that I was uncomfortable with my body. I didn't want him to see my bags.
>
> I was always a thong wearer before. I had a cute little body to go into my cute little underwear. Now he would see my granny pants.

The "granny pants" that Allis refers to are relatively high-waist underwear that has built-in pockets to support the pouches. They probably wouldn't differ dramatically from underwear that a lot of women wear, unless like Allis, they had a drawer full of sexy, lacy panties.

But having sex means the panties, whether they are pretty or ugly, have to get out of the way. Allis bought an ostomy belt, which both protects the bags and hides them. For anyone facing this challenge, we found that simply putting the term *sexy ostomy wear* into a search engine brings up lots of options—single ostomy, double ostomy, all sizes, all colors, custom made. Ready with her belt, she then outfitted herself for the big event: a black negligee. From the waist up and the pelvis down, she appeared to be presurgery Allis.

This first attempt at intimacy did not go as planned, however. They quickly realized that something was extremely different, and they didn't know how to work around it.

Allis had no vagina. A small amount of skin remained at the point of entry, but after that, the elastic muscular canal that serves such an important role in intercourse was gone. Were they aware of this—yes, but having a cognitive grasp that a pelvic exenteration removes the vagina and an intimate experience of what that means are two very different realities.

Relying on the "Ritual of 24 Hours" that had served her and her family so well before, Allis threw herself a pity party to mourn the loss of her vagina. Unfortunately, in the midst of this one, while she unleashed all of her emotions and tears, she plunged into a conversation she felt she needed to have with her husband.

Sobbing, Allis began with: "You have a wife who is forty-nine years old and has no vagina—no way to have normal sex. You don't deserve this. You need to be able to find somebody who can satisfy you because I can't."

He understood the sincerity of her message but seemed genuinely perplexed. "I don't love you just for your vagina," Craig said simply. "Do I miss that? Yes. But we can be creative and figure out other things to do."

And they did.

They got a lot of ideas from, as Allis calls them, "naughty stores," both online and physical ones. Although most of the sex toys they saw were more humorous than useful, they primarily saw value in them because they stimulated the imagination.

> I have to remember that a kiss goodbye or hello means a lot. We hold hands when we go out for a date night. I give him back rubs, and say things that I used to think, but now it seems important to actually say them, like "You sure are looking cute!" In fact, that one's become code for "I'm feeling a little frisky." And I make sure I prepare myself before

we get intimate so that I can have an orgasm, too . . . and when I do, it's very, very good.

A remaining side effect of the surgeries is some numbness of the labia, so Allis's preparation is taking a few extra moments to get herself completely ready mentally as well as physically. She not only wants to look as attractive as possible—for herself even more than for her husband—but also to have lubrication, a vibrator, and other helpful items at hand.

Allis and Craig have become completely familiar with what their bodies can and can't do together. They use their imagination to explore every possible way to enjoy their intimacy. Sometimes instead of aiming for sex, they enjoy a simple thrill like taking a ride in their Jeep and having the wind blow their hair back. The bottom line is that they have fun with the person each loves and trusts most in the world.

Allis did, of course, see her son graduate from high school. That was two years ago. She got what she wanted.

As a final note, Craig said,

> Her story is still going. She has used her disease to connect with others, help others, inspire others. Including me.
>
> People said to me, "What a terrible thing you're in!"
>
> Sure, it is terrible to watch someone you love go through this, and to go through it yourself. It's an ugly disease. But funny, at the same time, it led to beautiful things. We were deeply in love before—we were high school sweethearts—but we have grown together so much more.
>
> Allis has a saying that helps us stay on track, "You get to choose." So we choose to have a high-quality life.

II

OVERCOMING THE IMPACT

• 6 •

One Challenge at a Time

$\mathscr{T}$o begin the largely prescriptive section of the book, there is a close look at the psychosocial health challenges reported by woman after a cancer diagnosis:

- Sex was less enjoyable
- Frustration with sex life
- Feeling depressed
- Feeling less of a woman
- Worry about the future of their sex life

True stories in this chapter illuminate what incidents or confluence of factors mitigated those feelings. Again, meeting the challenges is not something the cancer patient does alone: There is a cadre of people in play here, both at home and in the clinical environment.

We have had many women tell us how they felt, what happened to make them feel different—better or worse—and what they would recommend to other women about healing their frustrations and concerns about their sex life. Those insights are featured throughout this part of the book.

SEX WAS LESS ENJOYABLE

Women in the UC study overwhelmingly reported that they found sex less pleasurable after the cancer diagnosis, and that included all types of sexual activity—oral, vaginal, and anal. It is not correct to assume, however, that lack of pleasure meant pain. Follow-up interviews pointed quite a bit to women withdrawing from pleasure; that is, they didn't commit to experiencing it. They expressed a sense that, for a while at least, they didn't feel they deserved to enjoy sex.

Immediately after treatment, Lily had an incredible amount of anger at the body changes that happened because of surgery. An ovarian cancer patient, she had an especially hard time emotionally and psychologically with the experience because of her body image. She had a huge incision from her breast bone to her pubic bone—seventeen or eighteen centimeters long, or about seven inches long. She was thin, a runner who was proud of her body. She found the combination of scarring and loss of her hair devastating to her self-image. While she was getting treatment, though, none of this mattered. She was in a fight to save her life and aesthetics had nothing to do with it. Afterward, however, she looked at herself in the mirror and said—in horror— "Where is my body?!? The body I worked so hard to keep healthy and beautiful is gone. The face is lined. The hair is gone. I have nothing left to show for all the work I've put into myself for thirty years."

As her body rehabilitated, as she grew her hair back and started to see and feel "herself," her desire came back fully. She told her oncologist that looking normal again made her feel like "a sexual person." This turned out to be an interesting gender identification issue. After her treatments, she felt "like a boy." The fullness of her breasts was gone due to weight loss from her inability to eat normally; that related to both treatments and stress related to the treatments. Her hair was gone due to chemotherapy. She had been thin, but without the muscle associated with running, she was just skinny, like a young teenage boy who'd had a growth spurt without the muscle to go with it.

At the time, she was in her late forties, so she had to deal with early menopause in addition to the body issues. Turning her sexual dysfunction around so she and her husband could enjoy sexual intimacy again took a year, but they did succeed. An important interim measure was addressing the psychological issues Lily had with her self-image. The effect of them bled into their relationship outside the bedroom—and a couple that has friction outside the bedroom usually has problems inside the bedroom as well.

Fortunately, Lily talked so much about looking like a boy and losing her body that her husband got the message. He paid attention to her efforts to enhance her feminine appearance and suggested they go out for dinner, for example, because she looked beautiful and he wanted to be seen with her. The combination of the visible signs of cancer treatment fading and her husband appearing delighted with the changes enabled them to get back on track sexually.

FRUSTRATION WITH SEX LIFE

The mechanical aspects of having sex are often the source of the greatest frustration. Ironically, some of them are the easiest issues to address. The next chapter contains numerous answers to the physical challenges of having more enjoyable sexual intimacy, from the medical (for example, Kegel exercises) to the nonmedical (for example, good lubricants). First and foremost, after going through surgery and other treatments, allow the body to heal. With one exception, the women we interviewed indicated they did not resume sexual relations with their partner for about three months after a hysterectomy or mastectomy. They added that, even then, it was not what they would call "normal," particularly if the surgery was followed by chemotherapy and/or radiation therapy.

Painful sex and *inorgasmia*, which is also referred to as *anorgasmia*, are the two frustrating problems that seem to surface the most. Physical therapists who specialize in pelvic floor therapy can often help a patient eliminate sexual pain. Again, the process is explored in some detail in chapter 7, which contains an entire section on "fixing the pelvic floor."

With inorgasmia, the woman either has difficulty achieving orgasm or never does. The surprise for women who finally talk about it after cancer treatment is that it's a common frustration that affects the majority of women! Take a look at the following four types of inorgasmia as described by *Consumer Health Digest*. Reflect on your own sex life as well as that of your female friends; the populations that can claim one or more of these types as true for them are quite large.

Types of Inorgasmia

- **Primary:** This means you have never experienced an orgasm in your life.
- **Secondary:** This means that you have experienced orgasms before but are now experiencing difficulty in reaching climax.
- **Situational:** This is when you are able to orgasm sometimes during certain situations like during manual stimulation or oral sex. This is the most common kind of inorgasmia experienced by women. In fact, most women are only able to orgasm when the clitoris is stimulated.
- **General:** This is when you are not able to achieve an orgasm in any kind of situation or with anyone.[1]

If your frustration is related to inorgasmia, and there is no environmental reason like medication or alcohol causing the problem, then you need to get to know your body better. You cannot expect your partner to guess what works, and you can't expect the frustration to be conquered with a hit-or-miss approach to either the clitoris or the G-spot.

One of our patients asked him pointedly after surgery: "Do I still have my G-spot?" Nothing had occurred in her therapy that would have caused it to go away. "Where is it exactly?" she asked. The answer is that it's near the top of the vagina on the front wall.

But after years of intercourse, some women still think the G-spot is like the Loch Ness monster: so elusive, it may be a myth. If you don't look for it, you won't know. And even if you can locate it, there is no guarantee that stimulation will cause an orgasm. For some women, focusing on the clitoris is the best way to go.

FEELING DEPRESSED

Depression is a huge risk factor after a cancer diagnosis, but as the treatments take their toll on appearance, energy, and mood, it can become a chronic issue.

Let's first get clear on what we mean by "depression" so that we don't confuse it with fleeting sadness, anxiety, or introspection. Andrew Solomon is a writer, lecturer, and professor of clinical psychology at Columbia University. When he talks about depression, he gives insights that are as much personal as they are clinical; he has suffered from severe depression. Here is how he describes the feeling that a dozen questions in the UC study approached from different angles:

> In 1991, I had a series of losses. My mother died, a relationship I'd been in ended, I moved back to the United States from some years abroad, and I got through all of those experiences intact.
>
> But in 1994, three years later, I found myself losing interest in almost everything. I didn't want to do any of the things I had previously wanted to do, and I didn't know why. The opposite of depression is not happiness, but vitality. And it was vitality that seemed to seep away from me in that moment. Everything there was to do seemed like too much work. I would come home and I would see the red light flashing on my answering machine, and instead of being thrilled to hear from my friends, I would think, "What a lot of people that is to have to call back." Or I would decide I should have lunch, and then I would think, but I'd have to get the food out and put it on a plate and cut it up and chew it and swallow it, and it felt to me like the Stations of the Cross.[2]

The study asked respondents to answer "yes" or "no" to this question both before and after the cancer diagnosis: "Have you often been bothered by little interest or pleasure in doing things?" This is precisely the lack of vitality to which Solomon refers. The unfortunate reality is that, if it were true before the diagnosis and treatment, then a series of traumas might give way to even more serious episodes.

But that's not necessarily so. Some patients give it a positive spin, saying that the diagnosis actually energized them. With their partners right beside them, they had a sense of purpose, a drive to fight and beat the disease. Now recall what we shared in chapter 3 about the aftermath of the fight. For a couple going through the cancer experience, suddenly there is a triggering event: The fight is officially over. No more treatments are on the horizon. All that's left is periodic follow-up visits with the doctor, and this is the time where a host of psychological and emotional issues can emerge with one of them being depression.

Intake interviews for cancer patients sometimes detect depression, so the team will watch for signs that it's worsening or not diminishing. The oncologist may initiate some kind of antidepressive therapy with the caveat that the patient meet with a mental health professional as soon as possible. As you might suspect, this is not uncommon in a cancer center. Anecdotally, we learned through interviews that major facilities will get about one patient a week who shows signs that she might be suicidal. In extreme situations, she would be sent immediately to the emergency department for a psychiatric evaluation.

The qualitative picture we got from combining study results with interviews is that roughly 80 percent of the gynecologic cancer patients who participated experienced what they would call depression for a brief period of time. More distressing is the fact that around 30 percent spoke of chronic depression.

We came across a particularly interesting explanation for the difference between at least some of the patients with ongoing depression and those whose depression was short-lived and mostly linked to the cancer diagnosis. The hypothesis is that the people with less or no depression were more capable of *positive illusions* than the depressed people. Barring anything organically amiss with them such as bipolar disorder, we might say that the latter group suffered from a relentless grasp of reality. The clinical name for it is *depressive realism.*

Shelley E. Taylor is a distinguished professor of psychology at the University of California, Los Angeles, who began her work around positive illusions by studying the coping process of breast cancer patients. Through interviews with them and their partners, she found that some of their beliefs relating to their chances for survival and health were, very simply, illusions. As a result, Taylor developed the theory of cognitive adaptation, which states that when someone faces a threatening event, her readjustment centers around finding meaning in her experience, gaining control over the situation, and boosting self-esteem.[3] Out of that came the more focused studies related to positive illusions.

Taylor concluded that these illusions promoted good health rather than undermined it. Some other social psychologists disagreed and said that their work showed that the positive-illusion people were actually maladjusted. But Taylor persisted in her work and amassed a body of evidence showing that cancer patients who harbored positive illusions had lower mortality rates than those without them. She has also been careful to note that useful self-aggrandizement, idealistic optimism, and exaggerated perceptions of control—the elements that constitute positive illusions—are not off-the-chart fantasies. In the conclusion to her study "Positive Illusions and Coping with Adversity," she and her teammate David Armor concluded: "Because positive illusions typically remain within modest bounds, and because people show a high degree of relative accuracy regarding their strengths and weaknesses, the 'illusion' component may be less consequential than some critics have suggested."[4]

One of the earlier studies that Taylor published about the topic has gained a kind of cult status. It provides a vivid illustration of how people with depression versus nondepressed people react to a simple video game. The two groups were asked to play a game in which they had to destroy monsters. At the end of the hour, the research team asked each group how many monsters they thought they had killed. Members of the depressive group were remarkably accurate, reporting a number within about 10 percent of the actual count. In contrast, the nondepressed people thought they had killed between fifteen and twenty times as many monsters as they had actually destroyed.

FEELING LESS OF A WOMAN

A uterus isn't very large—about the size of a fist. It's a bit mind-boggling to think that this relatively small thing that weighs less than half a pound can accommodate one or more babies. Yet for some women, the removal of this little organ that's even smaller than a heart can be a devastating event. If the breasts are the main external symbol of a woman's maternal nature, then the uterus is the internal symbol of it.

Some of the patients we interviewed did not feel particularly sexy after a hysterectomy; in fact, they felt like there was a hole in them—an empty space. There is no change in sensation related to this during an intimate encounter, so it isn't as though they or their partner would even notice. But if the woman senses a loss of her womanhood, then it can lead to sexual dysfunction. She might think, even subconsciously, "I'm not the woman I was." "I'm not the woman you married." Loss of breasts could logically have the same effect.

Compound that diminished sense of womanhood with chemo-caused baldness and a vagina constricted and dried out from radiation and you have a decidedly unsexy feeling. This is the source of the numbers from the study that overwhelmingly indicated that women who've experienced gynecologic cancers go through a period of feeling "less than."

Aside from healing so the visible signs of cancer treatments aren't obvious anymore, there are things a couple can do to restore the woman's sense of femaleness. We've stayed with some relatively generic insights here and reserved most of the specifics for the next chapter.

- Couples' activities that move you out of the routine in a long-term relationship can make you feel more like a woman. For example, one couple in which the woman was an endometrial cancer patient described strolling down the street of a city on the East Coast. There was a kind of Bohemian set of coffee shops, bistros, and clothing stores. One of the stores they passed had a sign indicating it featured lingerie. A block later, her husband asked her: "Do you want to see what they have?" "Sure, what the heck," she said. They walked in and were greeted by a clean-cut young man who invited them to browse as long as they liked. The shop did have some lovely lingerie in it, but the primary product offerings were an impressive collection of sex toys and videos. They stayed about fifteen minutes, bought nothing, but walked back to their hotel hand in hand.
- Use a calendar to your advantage. It's not a matter of exactly what you do as a couple as much as it is that the evening is special. Jeff and Joan were empty nesters who went through her treatments for ovarian cancer. While she was recovering from debilitating chemo treatments, Jeff had the bright idea to pick thirty-six days over the next year when they would do something special as a couple. "Joan, pick a number between one and thirty," he'd say. They repeated that until he had dates highlighted for the whole year when he would do something to show her what a great woman she was. One night, he invited her closest girlfriends over for a wine tasting. He disappeared for the evening, but she got quality time with friends that reminded her that, yes, she was one of the girls.
- Couples going through adversity like cancer want and need safety and security, which hopefully is intrinsic in their relationship. But let's look at Maslow's Hierarchy of Needs to see what else they might do to make a woman become more resilient in the face of a diminished sense of womanhood.

Maslow's Hierarchy puts physiological needs at the bottom, meaning that he sees the most fundamental needs of a human animal as food, clothing, and shelter. Above that is safety and security. Above that is love and belonging, a topic explored extensively in the "psychological/emotional solutions" section of chapter 7. The tier above that on the hierarchy is esteem; that is, feeling respected. After the blow to esteem presented by the invasion of a malignant tumor and the radical treatments to remove it, a woman needs respect in order to feel her womanhood.

WORRY ABOUT THE FUTURE

It's important to differentiate between the two types of worry when it comes to your sex life. This book focuses on physical intimacy, but as most human beings know, there is sex (vaginal, anal, and oral) without intimacy and intimacy without any type of sexual activity. We would ask you to consider that cutting out one and leaving the other—regardless of what gets cut—can still translate to sexual dysfunction. Not necessarily, but it can. Once you recognize that you are not quite balanced between them, it's a matter of determining whether or not you care enough to change that.

To begin the discussion, we want to give you three true stories with contrasts in the roles of sex and intimacy.

Intimacy Lost and Found

Within a month of relocating from New York to a midsized western town, Charlotte had a suspicion something was wrong with her. The first sign was a distended stomach. Half of her said, "You're forty now, so maybe your body is just losing its youthful look." The other half said, "Get it checked out."

Life intervened since she was just getting her children resettled in a new school. Besides, she had had a physical as well as a gynecological exam just before leaving New York, so she assumed if there were something wrong, a few weeks wouldn't matter much.

The symptoms mounted. Soon, she couldn't lie on her stomach, and she would feel full shortly into a meal. A tablespoon or two of food felt like a plateful. She had visible weight loss everywhere except her stomach.

Her new doctor tested her for H pylori, short for Helicobacter pylori, which is linked to chronic gastritis and gastric ulcers. The test came back negative, so Charlotte shared her suspicion that maybe it was fibroids. The next test was a CT scan.

The results came back a day before Thanksgiving. It was not a good holiday.

Her regular doctor referred her to a cancer center, where she had the CA 125 blood test. A normal result would be 35. Charlotte's was 4,000. She soon got confirmation that she had ovarian cancer. It had progressed to an advanced stage.

> I had to schedule surgery right away. I couldn't make my mind catch up with the world around me. Everything seemed to be whizzing by and I was screaming inside, "Wait, wait, wait! What's going to happen to my children?" I asked, "What's my prognosis?" but I knew I wouldn't be satisfied with anything less than, "Don't worry, Charlotte, we're going to cure you." Instead, she said, "It doesn't look good for you."

She had two children, ages eight and twelve, and a significant other, Keith, with whom she had just started sharing a home. They had gone together for six years, but the move out West enabled them to finally live together.

When she told Keith, she said she wasn't sure she could handle this fight. Since it was so bad, maybe she should just resign herself to dying.

"I'm going to do one of two things," he told her. "I'm either going to walk out of here and never come back because I am not going to watch you die, or you can fight. And if you fight, I'm right here."

Thinking that the greatest uncertainty was her survival and the greatest certainty was her relationship, Charlotte began the fight. She took every step with her sweetheart beside her—literally. Except for the three months when she was recovering from the surgery that cut her from sternum to pelvis, they didn't miss a beat with sex.

Charlotte's first move in taking control of her battle was switching physicians. She felt it was vital that a battle as tough as hers be waged with the help of someone she both respected and connected with. It gave her more optimism to be with her new doctor than she had felt since the diagnosis. Her confidence surged.

Still very groggy from the anesthesia, she was able to say hello to her surgeon—the one she had hand picked—in her room that evening. He smiled and said, "We have everything and it looks good." Then she fell asleep again. Waking up the next morning with more happiness than she'd felt in months, she realized it was her birthday. Unlike her Thanksgiving the previous year, it was a very good holiday.

When Charlotte decided she had a great chance of living a long life, she decided that chemotherapy involved a fashion statement. A beautiful black woman, she felt she could get away with headscarves and large earrings in a way that looked stylish—or she could go with a head of fuzz and earrings and still look chic. She told us, "I realized that if a white woman shaves her head, or wears a head scarf and big earrings, she just looks like a cancer patient with accessories!"

Through all of it, Keith was there. He paid the bills. He made sure the children were cared for when he took her to appointments. He was physically present, including showing desire for her at the worst of times. For a year and a half, he was Superman. They were both new in town, so there was rarely a backup. He couldn't take a weekend off and hang with the guys.

Charlotte's medical and logistical needs for eighteen months were relentless, and he took care of all of the logistical needs. And as far as their intimate relationship was concerned, Charlotte says, "It was a mental and emotional cyclone. We didn't have the best sex, but we still had it. We kept at it."

And then one day, Keith left for work and never came back. Charlotte knows he's alive because his sister told her that he's fine. He's a professional firefighter, so it was easy for him to relocate and quickly find work in another town.

There was nothing wrong with their sex drive and level of activity. Using nothing more than the nineteen-question Female Sexual Function Index (FSFI), they would score well—qualitatively not showing any signs of sexual dysfunction. Ultimately what they had, however, was sex without intimacy. That's a dysfunction of the heart.

Charlotte felt that Keith had done exactly what he said he would: be there for her the entire time she fought the disease. He kept his word, so she was able to forgive him. He'd had enough; he wanted an easier path now. The abrupt departure rattled her, though, and made her doubt that she was lovable.

She remained unsettled until, one Sunday, something odd happened— something that gave her an overwhelming sense of self-worth and direction.

One day I was sitting in church. My girlfriend had come from New York to visit me. I felt a push on my back, as though someone was touching me. In my head, I thought, I can see my girlfriend and the other people around me, and no one is touching me. The feeling got stronger, as though someone was pushing me to stand up.

The next thing I knew, I was talking. It's not like me to get up in front of people and speak. I had never done anything like this. I'm an intensely private person. There was no reason why I would stand up in church and tell my story. God doesn't give you an option to be selfish at a moment like that.

If you look at the Internet, if you look at the numbers, everything says I shouldn't be here. The numbers say I would have been gone a year by now. The things that should have happened, didn't.

My doctor put the numbers in my favor, and my God told me to tell people about my miracle.

In that moment, Charlotte experienced the kind of spiritual intimacy that helped her put her life with Keith into perspective. And it gave her a mission to help other women believe "they could come out on the other side."

RESTORING INTIMACY WITH THE HELP OF OTHERS

> We had a hard time. For months, I had to have an ostomy bag and at first it didn't fit well. You know what was literally coming out of my body! Before that, it was chemo and tubes attached to my body. None of this made me feel very attractive.

This is how Connie responded when we asked her how she regained her sex life with her wife, Jen. Recalling the revulsion she instinctively felt—revulsion mixed with empathy at seeing her partner suffer—Jen said, "Quite honestly, some of it was nauseating."

> Sex is one thing; intimacy is another. I knew that sex was out of the question for a while, but I would have enjoyed more intimacy. Just touching. But I think that Jen was freaked out in some ways.
>
> I'm a really strong person. I represent strength and getting through things to a lot of people—my spouse, my family, my friends—and that role tended to isolate me through much of my ordeal, which lasted more than a year. I had only one sister who came to visit me out of nine siblings. And most of them live within twenty-five miles. My best friend from college came to visit me and avoided the subject of my illness completely. I told her, "I don't want to talk about your son's little league team. I have cancer." She started to cry and admitted that she simply had not known how to handle the situation. I told her that we were in the same boat.

Her partner said, "She was going on with her life as though there was no bump in the road. Her family thought, 'Oh, it's Connie, she's fine.' She acted like everything was fine!"

> My one sister who came to visit me the few times I would let her also offered to go to chemo with me. Jen couldn't do it. It was too painful to see me sick and looking as though I might not be around tomorrow. But that didn't help me, know what I mean? I'm not needy; I just like affection.

And we did know exactly what she meant. She just wanted to feel closeness with the most important person in her life at a time when her mortality took center stage in her thoughts.

> I take care of myself. I went to therapy. I joined a support group. You can't talk about this with a lot of people. As much as they truly want to be there for you, they can't handle it.

As Connie's condition improved and her ostomy bag was removed, they were able to talk through it more, and be explicit about each other's needs. The hand holding, the soft touches, the kisses—they all followed eventually. Not immediately, but eventually. Connie's wise approach to restoring homeostasis in her life not only supported her health but also the health of her marriage.

INTIMACY WITH OR WITHOUT SEX

Toni and Dan retired at sixty-five, having both worked for different branches of the U.S. federal government for forty years. Suddenly, they were empty nesters with three grown children and good pensions, so a year later they moved from Washington, D.C., to the mountains of Colorado.

They embraced their new community and, over the next four years, grew to know just about everyone in town because of their volunteer work. They were healthy and relatively fit for their age. Toni had about thirty pounds she wished she didn't have, but life was good—until she noticed a dark discharge that she thought was incontinence. Immediately she went to her regular doctor who thought it might be an infection. Toni went home with an antibiotic cream that she thought was a necessary, messy inconvenience. "Why do I have to deal with this icky stuff now?" she thought. It was over the Easter holiday, and her three children and their spouses and children were all coming into town for meals, church services, and hikes in a national forest.

Easter Monday, Toni went back to her doctor, who tested her urine. Using her best medical jargon, she said, "Oh, there's all kinds of ugly junk in here." She prescribed another antibiotic for a urinary tract infection (UTI).

The following Friday, Toni got up during the night to go to the bathroom and bled all over the floor. It was worse than the worst period she'd ever had, and she'd stopped having those two decades before. Dan heard her shriek and jumped out of bed: "What shall we do?"

"If this doesn't stop in twenty minutes, we're going to the ER," she said.

Twenty minutes later, they got into the car and headed to the hospital. The doctor on duty gave her an order, "You must see Dr. J tomorrow." Dr. J was what everyone called the only gynecologist on staff at the hospital. He name was so long, everyone had given up trying to pronounce or spell it.

With the visit to Dr. J, a trek toward unprecedented human intimacy began for Toni and Dan. Surgery couldn't be scheduled for two weeks, so they went on a beach vacation during which, as Tony tells it, "We had an orgy." It wasn't really an orgy, but for a couple in their early seventies, it seemed like an orgy.

Her oncologist discovered during surgery that part of the uterine cancer had reached a Stage III level but had not spread to the lymph nodes. She was declared "clean" and scheduled for four sessions of radiation. Chemotherapy wasn't necessary.

We interviewed Toni and Dan three years after their experience, so they were now in their mid-seventies. Sitting with them together and listening to their story—they sometimes complete each other's sentences in a way that flows rather than interrupts—we picked up a sense of harmony. Dan said, "I didn't care about the sex. I just wanted Toni alive." Toni said, "We do all kinds of fun things together. Sex just doesn't happen to be one of them anymore!" And then they laughed.

For couples with emotional and psychological intimacy, their options on sexual intimacy are almost boundless. A strong bond between them suggests they maintain nourishing communication about all the topics that matter to them as a couple. Maybe their focus used to be on parenting and coordinating family schedules, but they evolved as their children grew. Now they talk more about moving toward a healthier lifestyle, or what a gripping television series they both enjoy. The point is that they communicate openly and regularly about issues of mutual interest and importance.

How much sex should a great couple like that have?

How much sex you have in your relationship is a negotiated element of it. There is no dysfunction if both members of the couple are happy with the level and style of intimacy they enjoy. Dysfunction comes into play when one person's pleasure—or comfort—is another person's physical or psychological/emotional pain.

Jenni Skyler, PhD, is a sex therapist who originated the term *Cheesecake of Pleasure* to describe the many sexually fulfilling options that a couple might explore in addition to intercourse. (We describe a sample cheesecake in chapter 8.) You can feel whole and close to another person, like Toni and Dan, without having the intercourse slice.

If you feel as though you want to have more sexual experiences of any kind, then aim for more. But if you feel neutral about it and enjoy the frequency of your sexual play as it is, then don't slap a "dysfunction" label on your love life just because you read something about what is "normal" or "average." You may want to have a session or two with a therapist to see if she or he can awaken new impulses and desires in you as a couple, but don't force it.

The closeness of holding hands, hugging, and cuddling is sufficient to release oxytocin, the hormone associated with love and trust. Couples with genuine intimacy can feel tightly bonded and even ecstatic in each other's company without ever having intercourse. They have a steady release of oxytocin as they enjoy other slices of the cheesecake.

· 7 ·

The Continuum of Solutions

- Medicine is a left-brained discipline; healing is a right-brained process.
- Healthy habits come from choices; physical well-being comes from feelings.
- Stress is vital to self-defense; stress is lethal to health and healing.
- Autonomy is vital for a human being; vulnerability is vital to connecting with another human being.
- Cars are built so they can be fixed; people are built so they can regenerate.

—Maryann Karinch and Trevor Crow,
Forging Healthy Connections:
How Relationships Fight Illness, Aging and Depression

There are physical and emotional/psychological solutions to overcoming sexual and marital dysfunction. Some of them are small actions, taken on a case-by-case basis, and some of them are pervasive in terms of lifestyle.

The solutions in this chapter fall into all three categories. Some are medical or scientific in nature, and some are nonmedical ones. Rather than simply lay out potentially helpful ways to transition from a lack of intimacy to intimacy, however, we want to start with *why*—why you really need to do this to improve your health.

Trevor Crow (Mullineaux) is the author of *Forging Healthy Connections*, and her area of concentration as a couples' counselor is Emotionally-Focused Therapy (EFT). Mullineaux's premise in her book is that we are built for relationships. The need for connection with other human beings is an intrinsic part of us and makes intimate relationships essential for health. She notes:

Our bodies thrive when we have great relationships. They suffer when we don't. The need for connection with other beings permeates the human body. Our bonds with other people profoundly affect our immune system—and we have a lot of science to back that up! In other words, relationships directly affect the mechanisms in our body that restore health and keep us healthy—and that make us sick. Health and healing benefit from positive thinking, but *thinking* isn't what sustains them—it's *feeling*. What gives our immune system juice is connecting intimately with another human being. The assumption that you are better off pursuing answers to *all* your problems intellectually is ruinous to relationships and to your health.[1]

As Mullineaux defines it, a healthy connection is a full-bodied experience. We are limited in our abilities to use emotion as a tool of healing and thriving if we think of it as just our brain's way of giving us a thumbs-up or thumbs-down signal on a particular interaction or event. Emotion happens throughout the body.

Perhaps one of the best explanations of this comes from Daniel Siegel, who talks about emotion as a verb instead of a noun in his essay "Emotion as Integration: A Possible Answer to the Question, What Is Emotion?" Siegel's essential message is, "Emotion-related words and concepts are active processes, not fixed entities. Seeing emotion as a verb opens our mind to a fluid, moving mechanism that acts, changes, transforms."[2] So, it might be more accurate to think of our feelings as blood circulating through the body rather than a sensation or judgment the brain sends to a body part like your tongue ("This crème brûlée makes me happy!") or your eyes ("I am so disappointed in this movie!").

If you want to give yourself an instant rush of full-bodied emotion, think back to a shocking or frightful moment in your life—one that charged up your sympathetic nervous system and put you on "red alert." You were driving on the highway and listening to the radio, and suddenly a police car sped closer and closer to you, lights flashing and sirens blaring. Your whole body screamed in anger and fear, "What did I do?" And then the police car sped past you and your whole body breathed a sigh of relief and felt happy that you had done nothing wrong. Your autonomic nervous system was at work, but there were emotions surging through you moment by moment.

There is more good news about intimate connection and its impact on human health. The act of actually connecting—that is, sexual relations—apparently has incredible health benefits. This is not a new concept, but one that is revisited time to time using the latest scientific testing methods.

On August 29, 2016, the world was once again buzzing with news about great sex (mostly between celebrities) when a report came out that sex is great—great for your health. Matt Tilley is a sex health expert on the faculty of health sciences at Australia's Curtin University. One of his areas of specialization is sexual dysfunctions, and he has uplifting findings about why it's worthwhile to take action to become sexually active and satisfied:

When we look at the function that those hormones might have then we can see that they assist to reduce stress, and of course endorphins specifically might act like a natural anti-depressant. . . . A regular sex experience with our partner that's positive, is going to facilitate a connection . . . we may have the function of oxytocin in there—or the love hormone as it's often referred to—which can help facilitate people's love and trust of one another.[3]

To extrapolate from Tilley's comments, you are physiologically better off trying to reap the immune system benefits of connection, as described by Trevor Crow Mullineaux, if you add actual sex to the mix. Tilley also notes that "sex and intimacy have been linked to self-esteem, feeling better about ourselves, and increased confidence."[4]

Now let's add another health benefit: When you have sex, your diastolic blood pressure decreases and your systolic blood pressure increases. That means that the pressure in the arteries when it is relaxing between beats goes down while the pressure in the arteries while the heart is beating goes up. So an abbreviated, overly dramatic, scientific explanation is that your risk of heart attack and stroke can go down. (Note that two of the primary ways to reduce your diastolic pressure are typically to exercise and manage stress, both of which may be accomplished by having sex.)

So if you combine the emotional, mental health, and immune system benefits of revving up your sexual activity, science is telling you to act now.

EMOTIONAL/PSYCHOLOGICAL SOLUTIONS

To learn tips about getting yourself in the mood for an intimate encounter and other psychosocial aspects of having sex, you can always read *Cosmopolitan*. (Really, do it.) Our solutions primarily address what needs to happen when you are still in a state of profound sexual dysfunction that has roots in psychological issues.

Even if you don't have serious problems but you want to elevate your conversations about sex and your full-bodied appreciation of holding hands—and everything else—then these insights will help you do that.

It's also important to mention that a positive feeling about your partner is fundamental to engendering greater intimacy. Lacking that—if you question the genuine caring of your partner, for example—then having sex will not deliver the emotional/psychological benefits addressed here. As we mentioned before in introducing the hormone oxytocin, it is released during all forms of intimate connection, but "intimate connection" obviously does not describe every sexual act. Just as your body sends you messages of trust and acceptance with the outpouring of oxytocin, it will also give you signals when trust is not authentic.

Talk Therapy

We heard from a number of female health care professionals who are in close contact with female cancer patients and with whom the patients share details of their sexual dysfunction. Whether the issue is psychological, such as self-esteem, or physical, such as painful dryness, they talk about the issue with another woman. When asked, "Have you discussed this with your husband?" the answer is often, "No! I can't do that."

That inability to have an open conversation signals a preexisting condition in the relationship. There was not conversational intimacy before, so why would it be any different now?

Trevor Mullineaux asserts that "now" is a lot different from "before"—that's why. Cancer changes your life, at least for a while. It doesn't have to be a completely negative event, but it is an important one. On the positive side for a relationship, cancer can present a life-changing opportunity to take your intimacy up a notch.

> Use cancer as an action-forcing event. Use it as an excuse to express your thoughts out loud to your partner: "I don't feel desirable right now. I've lost my mojo. But I still love you and I want you to love me. I need you." You make huge strides forward toward intimacy when you allow yourself to be vulnerable. You invite closeness and connection in a powerful way. You need that level of vulnerability to have a trusting, honest relationship with your partner—cancer or no cancer. Take advantage of the circumstances to make your marriage stronger and your quality of life better. Think of it this way: Cancer is part of your journey as a couple so make good choices about what that journey looks like.
>
> Any challenge in our lives has the potential to bring us to a higher state.[5]

In reflecting on how this plays out in the real world, Mullineaux relates the story of a couple that stopped seeing one of her colleagues after just two sessions. Five months after canceling an appointment, the husband called one day and said, "We just want you to know we think you're great, but we don't need you anymore." His wife had gotten uterine cancer and in the process of surgery, chemotherapy, and radiation, they had spent so much time together focused on healing, talking, and "looking on the bright side" that their relationship hit new heights. Two years later, they went back and told the therapist that they see their relationship in two major phases: "before cancer—when it sucked—and after cancer—when it's amazing."

Many couples do not have a success story like this, of course, and so their talk therapy may be the clinical kind that is focused on the sexual dysfunction undermining their relationship. Sex therapists might be psychiatrists, psychologists, or couples' counselors, but their commonality is training in the psychological treatment and rehabilitation methods that address sexual problems. As we indicated in chapter 4, a significant emotional source of dysfunction is stress. Sex therapists try to help reduce relationship stress by guiding couples toward more open communication about sexual wants and needs, for example. But what the sex therapist might also introduce that another counselor would not is "sensate focus exercises," which are intimacy exercises with their roots in the work of William Masters and Virginia Johnson. Sensate focus is, in fact, considered the centerpiece of Masters and Johnson's therapeutic work.

In a clinical setting, sensate focus essentially remains talk therapy, but it does involve physical homework for the couple. The aim of the exercises is to heighten the level of trust and intimacy that the couple feels with each other; the critical element is learning to give and receive pleasure. That's different from having sex with the goal of orgasm, where someone can end up reinforcing his or her own fear of failure.

The University of Notre Dame provides a handout, freely available online, on sensate focus. The following paragraph illuminates the purpose and value of the exercises:

> The problem attitude is that sexually you are going to try to make something happen—say, an orgasm—for your partner. However, this is just like trying to make your partner digest their food or fall asleep. You can't make any of these things happen, you can just get out of the way of it happening naturally. The alternative to this "touching to make something happen" attitude is "touching for your own interest." The best thing you can do for yourself and your partner is to be involved with your partner's body for YOUR interest. In fact, that's how most people start out thinking sexually. It is not selfish, because selfish would entail disregarding your partner's desires. You will care about your partner's desires, and your behavior will be within bounds your partner sets. However, you will not be trying to accomplish anything for your partner during your interactions. Your partner will actually enjoy being with you more if you enjoy it than if you were trying to do something specific to them.[6]

One of the benefits of sensate focus exercises would therefore be elimination of the fear of failure. Another would be exploiting the abundant nerve endings in the ears, lips, and inner thighs, parts that are largely ignored by vagina-focused couples. You might elicit some spine-tingling thrills just through exploratory touching that has no endgame in mind.

The therapist would offer ground rules and instructions for the couple attempting sensate focus exercises. In brief, they involve establishing a private erotic space they both like, removing distractions, and exploring through touch with no time pressure. Generally, breasts and genitals are off limits for the first few sessions, and talking is kept to a minimum unless one of the partners is uncomfortable. Another rule is "no agenda"; that is, neither person aims to elicit a sexual response. If it happens, that's great, but it is not planned.

Sex educator and relationship expert Yvonne K. Fulbright (*Touch Me There!*) offers this summary of the first four sessions of sensate focus exercises:

Session I:
Once your partner has assumed a comfortable position, begin by touching and stroking your lover's naked body for 10 minutes. As you work your way front and back, head to toe, use your enjoyment as a guide. As you touch your partner's figure, notice the texture, contours, warmth . . .
Now allow your partner to do the same to you, fully focusing on the sensations of being touched by your lover and your reactions to it. In either case, try to be as quiet as possible, so you do not take away from your awareness of physical sensations.

Take turns massaging each other for another 20 minutes each (in later sessions, this can include the breasts and groin).

Touch and explore your bodies at the same time for 20 minutes, focusing on the touch, not sexual excitement.

Session II:
Building upon the exercises of Session I, you are allowed to touch the breasts and genitals now. Start by touching other parts of your lover's body first, emphasizing physical sensations, before gradually working your way to the sex organs.

Take turns "hand-riding," a nonverbal technique where the partner being touched places his or her hand over the giver's to indicate the desired touch. This could be fast or slow, using more or less pressure, or moving to a different area. If needed, the receiver can explain desired touch. The giver should, however, still largely guide efforts.

Session III:
This stage is all about mutual touching, making the interaction more natural in the touch exchange. Simultaneous touch also allows partners to focus more on each person's body instead of paying attention to one's own response. Couples should communicate what they enjoy and want sexually, without getting caught up in the goal of achieving orgasm.

Session IV:
If the couple is dealing with a sexual disorder, they should work with a sex therapist to determine if more exercises are needed to focus on physical sensation. Lovers, however, will get to a point where they can proceed to full intercourse without any problems.[7]

Couples like Dan and Toni who no longer have a strong interest in intercourse could still enjoy sensate focus exercises as a way to amp up oxytocin production. Add some candles, a warm bath, and a good movie and you have a sensual mini vacation for a couple of any age.

If the exercises are done with a full commitment to the experience, there will be a level of comfort with physical closeness that supports deep trust. The couple will come to see vulnerability as a tool of intimacy.

Vulnerability as a Tool of Intimacy

Brené Brown is the guru of vulnerability. A professor at the University of Houston Graduate School of Social Work, she has conducted qualitative research about vulnerability for more than a dozen years. In other words, for all those years, she has collected stories about vulnerability and the related human behavior topics of courage, worthiness, and shame.

Early in her work, Brown was studying human connection and went around asking subjects about their experiences. Instead of hearing about connection, she generally heard about disconnection. Ultimately, she drew a conclusion: "The one thing that keeps us out of connection is the fear that we're not worthy of connection."[8] Wanting to understand that better, she focused on the interviews where people displayed a sense of worthiness; she wanted to know what those people had in common. Here's what she found—and what led her to a study of vulnerability:

Courage, specifically the courage to be imperfect. If you are reading this book and have experienced cancer, then ask yourself: Did you have one moment—even one—when cancer made you feel flawed? Having listened to countless cancer patients over the years, we would be amazed if we found one person who didn't feel damaged or diminished by cancer at any point in their experience with the disease. But we also found a great many who realized that cancer didn't make them "less than." These are the courageous patients who put cancer in its place as soon as possible. It's a lousy disease that is not an intrinsic part of you—not like your kindness, intelligence, sharp wit, or generous nature.

Compassion, which they showed themselves as well as other people. Recall the story of Allis and Craig featured in chapter 5. Allis gave great insight into her compassion for herself when she told us about her "Ritual of 24 Hours"; that is, the time she gave herself to be nuts after getting another horrible diagnosis or painful treatment. Whether consciously or subconsciously, she knew that the healthiest response to yet another traumatic event was to allow herself to be angry, sad, grieving, desperate, or whatever else she needed to be so she would be better equipped to return to her relationship with her family. She cared for herself, and that made it more possible for her to care for others.

Is it really so bad if you don't have compassion for yourself—if you consistently put other people first because that's what seems to come naturally to you? One result could be a potentially fatal condition called Takotsubo's cardiomyopathy—broken heart syndrome. It results from chronic stress in the aftermath of an emotional shock or trauma. If, like Allis, you had just gone through three rounds of cancer surgeries followed by multiple cycles of chemo and learned you were being hit once again with tumors, you would probably consider that a traumatic event. Allis allowed herself the time to respond and react any way she wanted to, and that helped her move past the trauma.

Flip that around and consider how much Craig could have been a candidate for broken heart syndrome if he did nothing but focus on the horror of another setback—if the only thing on his mind was Allis's pain, feelings, and needs. This is exactly what happened to elite open-water swimmer Lynne Cox, who was the first person to swim the Strait of Magellan and around the Cape of Good Hope. Her resting heart rate was normally 60 beats per minute, but she began experiencing episodes of erratic, rapid heart rates, with her resting heart rate even hitting 157 beats per minute. It began happening after decades of taking care of seriously ill parents, and then having her beloved yellow Labrador die right after her parents died. With her parents, she had been by their side with both emotional and physical support for twenty-five years. In an interview with Robin Young on WBUR/NPR's *Here and Now*, Cox said, "To have my folks and my dog pass, it was like everything in my world was going away."[9] Fortunately, it is possible to recover fully from broken heart syndrome—but you have to show compassion for yourself and to commit to destressing behaviors.

Craig did something for himself—possibly averting a severe health threat like Takotsubo's cardiomyopathy—that parallels a destressing behavior Lynne Cox adopted to counter her heart problem. She was a swimmer who temporarily couldn't swim because she was so sick. One day, she filled a deep sink with water and started moving her hands through it. Then she put on her cap and goggles, and "suddenly felt that aliveness that you feel when you're doing something you just love."[10] Doing that gave her pleasure and hope as well as the title for her memoir, *Swimming in the Sink: An Episode of the Heart*. Craig started to play guitar, mandolin, and other string instruments again. It not only effectively destressed him but it also brought the joy of music back into the lives of Allis and Craig. Like Cox's swimming in the sink, it helped give them pleasure and hope.

Connection "as a result of authenticity," explains Brown. "They were willing to let go of who they thought they should be in order to be who they were."[11] Jason was the hard-charging pastor of a growing church when his wife got sick. His immediate impulse was to draw down his workload and focus on her. But it seemed as though he was even busier at the church and getting praise from his congregation about his abundant energy both to care for his wife and to meet the ministerial needs of church members. He was amazing! Unfortunately, the man his wife needed didn't really feel amazing, and he was not being true to himself or to his relationship with her. More than cancer, this sustained pretense set in place a chronic dysfunction in their relationship.

Vulnerability as a necessary element in a quality life; for example, the willingness to be the first to say, "I love you." A person who embraces vulnerability knows that saying "You're my best friend!" or "I love you" doesn't involve a guarantee that the other person feels the same way or will respond in kind. It means there is no regret in expressing that kind of genuine feeling.

In modern society, practicing vulnerability seems antithetical to most of us because we feel we must have our emotional armor on or we will suffer too much. One of the most touching aspects of the interview with Craig was how he realized that his initial response to Allis's many cancers was to be her "one-through-ten" source of toughness. But that approach fell far short. In Craig's case, when he allowed himself to say, "I need help" and he found that help in his relationship with Allis, his family, and his God, he embraced vulnerability. It was through vulnerability that he developed genuine strength.

In chapter 4, we looked at moments and events during the cancer experience when a woman is likely to feel violated; some women have even said it's like being raped. A normal response to that feeling is to harbor the commitment, "I will never be hurt again!" In some ways, it's like a woman whose husband has an affair. Even though they go to marriage counseling, she consistently tells herself, "I will never be hurt again!"

Well, you may get rid of the cancer and you may have a husband who is remorseful over the affair and will never do it again, but if you hang on to "I will never be hurt again!" as a mantra, you also won't ever be happy again. You have to know what hurt feels like in order to feel the comfort of intimacy and love. You need vulnerability.

Vulnerability is a deeply human ability that only really courageous people who love themselves can have. With cancer, you are threatened by a lot of external sources, but when you face that with your partner, admitting that you not only want to be with each other but also *need* to be with each other, then your connection grows more intimate. To need someone is not the same as being needy; it just means that you consider that person an essential part of your life, happiness, and health.

In terms of your conversations about sex, vulnerability will serve you well in that as well. Go ahead: Be the first one to say, "Let's try this . . ."

THE POWER OF THANK YOU

When Jay started seeing Cara, he told her that feeling appreciated was really important to him. Cara heard him, loud and clear.

Five years into their marriage, she developed ovarian cancer. She was a personal trainer, so her body awareness was very high and the cancer was diagnosed earlier than is the case with most ovarian cancer patients. Nevertheless, the surgery meant a loss of natural lubrication, among other changes that would affect their sex life.

Jay spent the night in her room after her surgery. He accompanied her to all the follow-up appointments. He surprised her with flowers throughout her recovery period. He bought her a gorgeous wig when her hair fell out after chemo. And on and on.

Each and every time Jay did something kind for Cara, she thanked him . . . and she wrote him a little note. After the surgery, she wrote it on a square of the paper placemat on her dinner tray. After that, she wrote cards or scrawled "thank you" on a balloon.

Jay needed to hear and see appreciation; Cara's expressions of gratitude made him feel loved as well as thanked. His need was not unusual.

In her unusually short three-minute TED Talk, "Remember to Say Thank You," counselor Laura Trice explains that people are wise to tell their loved ones how they need to feel appreciated.[12] And their loved ones are wise to pay attention and deliver the goods. This isn't hard, and it doesn't exactly necessitate counseling with a PhD therapist. But it can be one of the keys to intimacy that elevates day-to-day enjoyment of the relationship.

REVVING THE MENTAL MOTOR

Two interrelated facts help us grasp the "why" and "how" of getting in the mood for sex. First, for a committed couple, great sex is premeditated. Second, it's common knowledge, or should be, that foreplay helps a woman heat up for sex.

Planning

Psychotherapist Esther Perel is an expert on sexuality and is most known for her concept of erotic intelligence, popularized by her best-selling book *Mating in Captivity: Unlocking Erotic Intelligence*. In her TED Talk, "The Secret to Desire in a Long-Term Relationship," Perel asserts that couples who have been together for years and are still in a passionate relationship don't fool themselves into thinking that the spontaneous sex they had on their third date is something to aim for. Even if we put aside the physical challenges to spontaneous sex that come with age, such as dryness for a woman and difficulty with erections for a man, there are powerful reasons for couples to plan their sexual encounters. Perel explains:

> Erotic couples understand that passion waxes and wanes. It's pretty much like the moon. It has intermittent eclipses. But what they know is they know how to resurrect it. They know how to bring it back. And they know how to bring it back because they have demystified one big myth, which is the myth of spontaneity, which is that it's just going to fall from heaven while you're folding the laundry like a *deus ex machina*, and in fact they understood that whatever is going to just happen in a long-term relationship, already has.
>
> Committed sex is premeditated sex. It's willful. It's intentional. It's focus and presence.[13]

Perel also has something to say about the key ingredients of planning for good sex; namely, imagination, playfulness, novelty, curiosity, and mystery. Couples who have been together for a while tend to have, and regularly rely on, the key ingredients of a committed relationship on a daily basis. They can depend on each other, feel safe with one another, and predict accurately how the other person will respond in a given situation. That's not very exciting, is it? In order to spark desire, you need just the opposite. You need a taste of risk and adventure, titillating surprises, novelty—the kinds of experiences that your imagination conjures up. And when imagination flavors planning, then "planning" doesn't sound like such a boring, anticlimactic word.

Foreplay

You don't have to seek out age-restricted videos on YouTube to get affirmation of the value of foreplay. Even WebMD offers a jaunty article on the importance of it in which the 4'7" giant of sexual information, Dr. Ruth Westheimer, asserts, "It's particularly important for women to have successful foreplay because it takes a woman a longer time [than a man] to get up to the level of arousal needed to orgasm."[14]

Physical elements of foreplay, some of which are addressed later in the chapter, are rather codified in comparison to the mental ones. Certain actions tend to work well with most women. It's a bit different with the mental aspect of foreplay, however. What mentally contributes to arousal for women runs a broad spectrum.

One exception to this is genuine compliments. The women we interviewed agreed that a mental aspect of foreplay they find essential is some expression by a partner that they are desirable. The "ick factor" with cancer and its treatments invariably leaves women feeling less attractive than they might have felt in the past. The partner needs to give audible, as well as visible and kinesthetic, cues that the body he (or she) is about to make love with is a body he *wants* to make love with. He doesn't look at you and see drainage tubes coming out of your chest area or a sternum-to-pelvis incision. He looks at you as a beautiful woman who is, thank heavens, alive and in love with him.

To illustrate the point that mental stimulation can come from radically different sources for different women, consider these conflicting reviews from female readers on Amazon.com of *Fifty Shades of Grey* (Book I):

> This reader gave it the top rating of five stars—"Lots of anticipation and romantic sexiness."

> This one gave it one star, probably because zero is not an option—"I enjoy erotica and heard so much about this book that I had to give it a shot, but I'm five chapters in and just can't take it anymore."

In asking, "What movies do you find erotic?" we heard praise from one woman for the 2003 Bernardo Bertolucci film *The Dreamers*, while another woman said *The Dreamers* was so boring that she and her husband turned it off to watch the news.

Clearly, then, finding out what stimulates you or your partner might involve conversation and experimentation if this is going to be foreplay that is successful for both of you. The alternative, of course, is finding something that you alone enjoy and indulging in it before a sexual encounter with your partner.

After Allis's major surgery to remove every "female organ," she was left with no vagina and slight nerve damage to her clitoris—unavoidable results of the surgery that most certainly saved her life. She admitted that erotic literature began to play a role in her preparation for sex. Having her mind fully committed to the experience enhanced her pleasure and made it easier for her to climax. Realizing that, and acting on it, was an enormous boost to Craig's satisfaction as well. As a number of partners told us, they needed their wife or girlfriend to enjoy sex fully, otherwise they'd feel like a user or abuser. One husband went so far as to say that, before his wife started enjoying sex again, he felt like a pervert.

Invest some time in doing self-examination of what your brain perceives as erotic. Does a, b, or c below suggest eroticism to you—or are you more aroused by a spat between members of Congress on CSPAN?

a. "I comply, and he drags me down the bed so that my arms are stretched out and almost straining at the cuffs. Holy cow, I cannot move my arms." (E. L. James, *Fifty Shades of Grey*)

b. "You should be kissed and often, and by someone who knows how." (Margaret Mitchell, *Gone with the Wind*)

c. "While I've been naked before, I've never been bare. Not like I am with him. I feel like he can see every bit of me, every ugly, unlovable part of me I've tried for years to hide away. He sees me. And he wants me anyway." (Brighton Walsh, *Caged in Winter*)

As part of the mental preparation for sex, many experts recommend some kind of ritual before and after having sex. One of the simplest is to hold hands.

Holding Hands and Other Brain Tricks

Holding hands has been scientifically proven to reduce stress, which means it's a perfect prelude to sex. As we noted in chapter 4, activating the parasympathetic nervous system is step one in moving toward a satisfying intimate encounter.

University of Virginia psychologist James Coan published a study called "I Want Need to Hold Your Hand: The Social Regulation of Emotion" in the journal *Psychological Science* in 2006. The study documented the effect that holding hands had in diminishing a fear response. Using functional Magnetic Resonance Imaging (fMRI), Coan monitored the responses of sixteen married women when he administered small electric shocks every time they saw an "X" flash before their eyes. When the women were alone, their brains lit up when they felt the shock. When a stranger held their hand during the experiment, there was a noticeable decrease in the shock response. When holding the hand of their husband, the shock response plummeted. Of the sixteen women, those in the happiest relationships felt the most relief.[15] This is an example of using a connection with another person to engage the parasympathetic nervous system. EFT couples' counselors like Trevor Crow Mullineaux refer to this as coregulation, which is a therapeutic technique used to help couples understand the visceral power of connection.

Coan built on his work in the arena of human connection to develop his Social Baseline Model, which proposes that people are hard-wired to maintain close proximity to other humans as part of a strategy to reduce energy expenditure relative to energy consumption.[16] That means our bodies work harder when we tackle something alone—and that includes healing. One experiment that illustrates his theory involves putting a heavy backpack on a person standing alone at the base of a hill. Coan would ask, "How steep do you think the hill is?" and the person might say something like "forty-five degrees." Coan would then introduce another individual to the scenario and have him simply stand beside the person with the backpack. The scenario presented is that they would climb the hill together. What this repeatedly did was reduce the first person's perception of how steep the hill was. Instead of forty-five degrees, he might change his mind when asked again and say it's more like a thirty- or twenty-degree incline. When the person with the backpack thinks the hill is steeper, it requires more motivation to climb it; the brain is in overdrive trying to get the body ready to take on the challenge. Mullineaux explains the relevance to our most intimate relationship this way:

> Our brains are particularly sensitive to the load-sharing significance of our loving connections. People in trusted relationships will invest less effort in their negative impulses, leaving them less reactive to threat cues and other signs of possible harm. So, we are wired to outsource some of the things that occupy our minds to those with whom we have close relationships. A practical result is that our brains use less energy.[17]

In the context of the cancer experience, this means the connection we have with our partner enables us to devote more energy to healing—which accelerates the time it takes for us to physically regain sexual functioning.

The final note in this section on engaging the brain to support sexual functioning is more aimed at the male partner than the female reader. In the Esther Perel TED Talk about desire that is referenced above, she makes the point that erotic couples "understand that foreplay is not something you do five minutes before the real thing. Foreplay pretty much starts at the end of the previous orgasm."[18] In other words, it's an ongoing activity that keeps the mind circling back to the joy of connecting. Simple things like sending a loving text like "I miss you already," calling with a funny story, or taking three seconds to share a kiss before you take out the trash sends the message that your life together has quality and spunk—and that you are looking forward, not backward.

And as a couple, what you might want to do is keep a bucket list related to sexual play that each of you adds to on a regular basis. As Perel would recommend, keeping imagination in the game is an essential part of sparking desire.

PHYSICAL SOLUTIONS

In this section, we address both medical and nonmedical approaches to sexual health, with some of the nonmedical ones being essential to improved sexual functioning after treatment for a gynecologic cancer. It's not as though the information is irrelevant for a noncancer population, but this guidance addresses issues that a great many gynecologic (and breast) cancer patients have introduced into the conversation with health care professionals.

Keep in mind that a lot of our human sexual response is geared on muscle contractions and relaxation. We often think of nerves and the sensations they pick up as the source of pleasure, but without the muscles functioning in conjunction with the experience of that pleasure, we can't have full-bodied climax.

Fixing the Pelvic Floor Muscles

Julia Bunning, PT, DPT, specializes in helping patients with pelvic floor muscle dysfunction. Women who experience pain during intercourse, have postoperative pain, and are plagued with incontinence, constipation, and pelvic organ prolapse are just a few of the types of patients who come to her for pelvic floor therapy. The pelvic floor is a network of muscles, ligaments, and tissues that act like a hammock to support the uterus, vagina, bladder, urethra, and rectum—the structures within the pelvis. Unlike the other discussions so far of this region of the body, the focus in physical therapy rehab is on the musculoskeletal system. Physical therapists who treat the pelvic floor are often referred to as "women's health" physical therapists (or "men's health"). While Bunning stresses the importance of the initial subjective interview during her evaluation, she also conducts an assessment of the pelvic floor muscles. Bunning's internal and external exams of patients' muscles enable her to determine if the muscles are functioning normally. She assesses the muscles' strength, endurance, and coordination—that is, if they can both contract (or shorten) and relax (or lengthen). In the pain population, a common problem is that the pelvic floor muscles are overactive or chronically in a shortened position. This can lead to impaired ability to contract the muscles and increase the risk of incontinence, for example.

Another issue some women have is lack of muscle coordination. Bunning explains, "Sometimes we ask our patients to contract their vaginal muscles and instead of contracting they bear down or strain, elongating the muscles. Sometimes they do not have the body awareness to know how to contract."[19] Poor coordination of pelvic floor muscles may contribute to bladder dysfunction or incontinence, worsening prolapse, and/or pelvic pain.

A study involving forty-seven women with a pelvic dysfunction resulting in incontinence illustrated the problem dramatically. "Assessment of Kegel pelvic muscle exercise performance after brief verbal instruction" sought to determine if women given verbal instructions on performing Kegel pelvic muscle contractions would do them correctly. The study found that 49 percent had an ideal Kegel effort, but 25 percent displayed a Kegel technique that could actually worsen the incontinence.[20]

This is why Bunning's starting point in therapy is patient education. She wants to ensure, to whatever extent possible, that the person with pelvic dysfunction understands the anatomy and physiology contributing to their dysfunction, as well as the body mechanics of what's gone wrong and what can be done to address the problem rather than exacerbate it. A physical therapist can also do an exam to verify that the exercises are being done properly.

With surgery for any gynecologic cancer, one or more pelvic organs might be removed, or a portion of an organ might be removed. They are all rather close together, so taking an organ out can increase the risk for prolapse, or slipping forward or down of part of another organ. So if the cervix is removed, for example, it's possible that the bladder would fall down a bit. A physician would diagnose the prolapse and then may send the patient for physical therapy to try to restore muscle integrity in the area. Strengthening pelvic floor muscles won't "cure" the prolapse because it's a problem related to an organ, but it can mitigate the symptoms of falling out and downward pressure.

It is well worth it to find out if you are contracting your pelvic floor muscles correctly because Kegels can contribute a great deal to sexual satisfaction. In terms of restoring sexual functioning, Memorial Sloan Kettering Cancer Center indicates that Kegel exercises can help improve women's sexual health and pleasure by:

- Relaxing the vaginal muscles, allowing the vagina to be more open. This is helpful for women who experience pain during sexual intercourse and/or with pelvic exams.
- Increasing sexual arousal.
- Improving a woman's ability to reach orgasm.
- Improving blood circulation to the vagina.
- Increasing vaginal tone and lubrication[21].

Regarding the first point, the narrowing of the vagina—or stenosis—is something we've discussed earlier in the book as a side effect of vaginal brachytherapy. Kegels alone are not enough in the aftermath of radiation. Whether or not the patient goes to a rehabilitation facility for therapy to address the issue, regular dilation for about six months is a must.

But aside from radiation as a triggering event for vaginal narrowing, the cancer experience can lead to so much stress in a person's life that the patient might place that stress in the pelvic area. Consider how common it is for people to hold stress in their shoulders and neck. Similarly, some women hold their tension in their pelvic floor. Chronic tightening or holding tension in the pelvic floor muscles can lead to pelvic pain. For people who have had chronic pain, muscle "guarding" is a common occurrence. For the pelvic population, this chronic "guarding" or tightening can exacerbate pelvic pain and cause the muscles to be in spasm. An obvious result would be painful intercourse. Either initial penetration or deep thrusting—or both—could cause the woman tremendous pain.

If the problem is with the introitus, or entrance to the vagina, penetration may not even be possible. The answer may be a set of dilators, starting with one that is about the size of a finger and moving up in progressively greater diameters. If the pain occurs with deep thrusting, then possible "overactivity" or tightness of the deep pelvic floor muscles may be causing the pain. Sometimes, Bunning also recommends a low-frequency vibrating dilator. Just as a gentle vibration would relieve tense muscles in your back and shoulders, the same can be said for the benefits to the pelvic floor of a vibrator. She cautions that use of vibration is not appropriate for all patients, and that when it is appropriate it should be a lower-frequency as opposed to the high-frequency vibration, which may promote stimulation. Stimulation or high-frequency vibration is the opposite reaction from the desired one; that is, it could create more guarding or orgasm, and therefore, more tension or muscle spasm.

When your dysfunction is caused by tight, deep muscles, orgasm can be painful. When you have an orgasm those pelvic floor muscles are contracting and going into spasm. If they are already in spasm—and they don't know how to "let go"—then orgasm can deliver more pain than pleasure. The aim of down-training the pelvic floor is to learn how to release tight muscles, improve coordination, and relax the pelvic floor.

Lisa M. Ruppert, MD, is a physician of physical medicine and rehabilitation, also known as physiatry, who specializes in evaluating cancer patients and cancer survivors who have neurological and musculoskeletal impairments related to their cancer and its treatment. Sexual dysfunction is among her particular clinical interests.

In her practice at Memorial Sloan Kettering Cancer Center, she works with a multidisciplinary approach to rehabilitation. Ruppert's team includes a sexual health psychologist, a nurse practitioner specializing in women's health, and a physical therapist who, like Julia Bunning, specializes in pelvic floor rehabilitation. Her first step in managing these patients includes a thorough history and physical examination. This allows patients to discuss their symptoms in length and to determine the underlying etiology of symptoms. Examination includes an assessment of sensation, strength, and reflexes in the lower extremities and assessment of tissue quality and pelvic anatomy and the pelvic floor muscle, including sphincter function. An assessment of available imaging is also included in this step and further helps determine a diagnosis.

Ruppert talked about the importance of focusing on muscle control and bowel and bladder management in terms of sexual dysfunction. Muscles and nerves involved in the bowel and bladder also play a role in the sexual response cycle. She mentioned an example of a patient whose underlying dysfunction stemmed from a spinal cord injury.

> I cared for a patient with gyn cancer and spinal cord involvement from metastatic disease. She struggled with emptying her bowel and bladder and noted incontinence episodes with orgasm. These incontinence episodes made her reluctant to engage in intercourse with her husband. Our starting point in management was establishing a bowel and bladder program that she could not only perform daily but prior to intercourse. These programs included medication management, emptying strategies including double void and Crede, and pelvic floor therapy for sensory retraining and muscle coordination.[22]

Double voiding is a bladder-training technique to help patients eliminate urine completely from the bladder. Upon the sensation of complete emptying, an individual stands and sits back down with the goal of emptying any remaining urine. Another technique is the Crede maneuver in which a patient places extrinsic pressure in the suprapubic region to assist with elimination. One trick to get the pelvic floor muscles to relax is to keep an inward curve in the lower back and letting the lower abdominal wall relax forward. This can be accomplished by the use of a step stool when toileting.[23]

With some surgeries, there is a lot of scar tissue that affects the pelvic muscles' ability to contract and relax during emptying as well as intercourse. Part of the assessment by the therapist, therefore, is finding how much of that condition is coming into play. Therapists will often try to break up the scar tissue with manual therapy. There is more about the value and technique of breaking up scar tissue in the section below on rehab after breast cancer surgery, but in this case, the thing to note is that the therapist is focused on the perineum; that is, the area between the anus and the vulva (in a man, it's the scrotum).

Unlike double voiding, many of the therapies involving the pelvic floor are a lifelong commitment. To keep yourself healthy and satisfied, you want to keep doing your exercises on a regular basis.

WHAT NERVE(S) YOU HAVE BELOW THE BELT

The two areas of focus here are the pudendal nerve and the complementary relationship between the sympathetic and parasympathetic autonomic nervous systems. And with "autonomic," think "involuntary" or "automatic."

Pudendal Nerve

At the end of the last subsection, we brought the perineum into the conversation. The pudendal nerve is the main nerve of this part of the body. The pudendal nerve branches into three smaller ones. To give an overview of their areas of operation, we would say that one affects the anal canal, rectum, and skin in that area; another one, called the perineal nerve, is involved with vagina, urethra, and labia in women and the scrotum in men; and the third is the dorsal nerve of the clitoris in women and the penis in men. In short, the pudendal nerve is important for sexual function because it carries signals to and from the genitals, area around the anus, and urethra.

So in addition to musculoskeletal problems, scarring, and psychological issues as possible causes of sexual dysfunction, another possibility in play is damage to the pudendal nerve. It could not only affect how much a person feels but also how much sensory feedback is going up the spinal cord to the brain. Sexual response can therefore become rather unpredictable.

Pudendal nerve damage could be one of those preexisting conditions that the patient was unaware of until she entered rehab after cancer surgery. Trauma to the pelvic area during childbirth or riding a bicycle frequently are two of the potential causes of pudendal nerve damage in addition to surgery in the pelvic region.

There are other nerves and other types of nerve damage that can affect sexual functioning, of course, but the pudendal would automatically receive focus by physiatrists like Ruppert helping a woman after gynecologic cancer surgery. According to the Health Organization for Pudendal Education, treatment options include lifestyle changes, physical therapy, medication management, botox, pudendal nerve blocks, pudendal nerve decompression surgery, and neuromodulation.[24] Regarding the last option, neuromodulation is a way to counteract pain that is "felt," but it's essentially a phantom pain.

Sympathetic and Parasympathetic Systems

The nervous system of the body is divided into two large categories of function. We might broadly characterize them as "up" and "down"

—sympathetic and parasympathetic, respectively—with each having a critical role in our ability to function on a day-to-day basis.

We introduced these two parts of the autonomic nervous system and their relationship to the sexual response cycle in chapter 4 by citing the words and research of stress expert Robert Sapolsky. As a reminder, your sympathetic nervous system kicks in when you perceive danger or are in a state of heightened excitement. Your breath quickens, your heart rate accelerates, blood flows to your muscles, and other advantageous changes automatically occur to prepare you for action. The parasympathetic system is the opposite of that in some key ways; we prefer to call it complementary rather than opposite, though, because you need both. You can't be on red alert all the time or your immune system will collapse, among other things. You need the effect of the parasympathetic to help you relax, digest your food, and have proper reproductive functioning.

Sex is the interplay of both systems. Arousal is mediated by the sympathetic nervous system. You are anticipating a very physical act, so you are revving up. The parasympathetic nervous system, however, works to make sex pleasurable in many ways. If the sympathetic gets you into the moment, the parasympathetic makes the moment feel good. Thank the latter for your vaginal lubrication and the vagina dilating and becoming more elastic. Orgasm and ejaculation are mediated by the parasympathetic nervous system. Again, we call your attention to Sapolsky's entertaining explanation of the interplay that we cited earlier.

Damage to the nervous system chain can occur as a result of surgery, chemo, radiation, and other components of the cancer experience. The fibers for these systems are called ganglia, located along the spinal cord. A spinal injury could therefore affect them, but so could any cancer treatment that affects the efficiency of the ganglia. The brain won't get the message that something is supposed to be pleasurable, for example.

Many patients who have chemotherapy get taxol, a substance originally extracted from the bark of a yew tree. (Those who think of chemo as nothing but synthetic poisons might consider the origin of this medicine, one of those on the World Health Organization's List of Essential Medicines; that is, it's fundamental in a basic health system.) Unfortunately, neuropathy is a potential side effect of taxol, so the patient might have tingling and/or loss of sensation in certain areas of the body. It's caused by the active agent in taxol, which gets deposited in the nerve ganglia and reduces their functioning. The downside of this amazingly effective medicine, therefore, is sometimes that sex is not as pleasurable while the nerves are "clogged" by the taxol. Taxol is not the only substance that puts the patient at risk for neuropathy, but it is a prime offender.

The accumulation of the deposits corresponds to how much chemotherapy the patient has received as well as certain characteristics of the patient herself. Three rounds of chemo might not result in any effects, but nine rounds of chemo would likely create a noticeable impact on sensation. Some patients might have unnoticeable effects, whereas others find the tingling and numbness a long-term haunting effect of treatment.

In most cases, the effect goes away after about six to nine months because the patient's metabolism pushes it out of her system. But there are cases in which the damage is permanent.

Trying to pinpoint research-based evidence of what might counter the nerve-damaging effects of taxol and other chemotherapy medicines is frustrating. Anecdotally, some patients have noticed improvement by taking Vitamin B6 regularly. This is a vitamin that had a demonstrated role in cognitive function, so their experience with sharpening nerve sensitivity makes sense. But we have to emphasize that any evidence that it helps counter chemo-caused neuropathy is anecdotal. Another caution we would offer—from personal experience—is that dosage of B6 is important. Taking too much will create a short-term "hot flash" that is quite uncomfortable.

There are also pharmaceutical ways to address the problem of nerve tingling or pain, such as gabapentin, originally used as an antiepileptic medication to counter convulsions. It affects biochemistry and nerves that cause pain as well as seizures. Unfortunately, it makes some people drowsy, so this is a drug that wouldn't seem to go well with sexual intimacy. On the positive side, the prescribed length of time to take a drug like this to counter neuropathy is brief.

There are also devices that integrative medicine experts suggest *might* be helpful, such as the TENS unit, or Transcutaneous Electrical Nerve Stimulation device. Many people who have gone through surgery of different kinds—think a college football quarterback who had to have knee surgery after a lateral hit—have used a TENS unit to expedite healing. Its job is to cause muscle contractions with the intended result of increased blood flow through the small blood vessels in the muscle tissue.

You don't want nerve damage of any kind. If you think you've lost some sensation, discuss this with your doctor, a nurse, your support group, and with a physical therapist. Speak up about what hurts or what you don't feel at all, even if someone says it shouldn't hurt or lacking sensations is normal. If you hear, "Now you should be feeling this . . . " and you don't feel it, speak up!

REHAB AFTER BREAST SURGERY

Impaired range of motion and abnormal posture are functional impairments that physiatrists, such as Ruppert, address in patients post breast cancer surgery, and even throughout the time when the patient is getting adjusted to the permanent implants. Shoulder range of motion and back posturing are primary areas of focus in rehab.

In tackling range-of-motion problems in the shoulder, it's essential to do it with someone who knows how breast surgery affects the body. The trauma of surgery to the pectoral area is what causes the range-of-motion issues because the pectoral muscles are involved in the shoulder girdle. They connect the front walls of the chest with the bones of the upper arm. One possibility is that the surgery can lead to scar tissue that pulls the humeral head—the top of the long bone at the upper part of the body—toward the front of the body. A therapist who primarily works with people injured in the gym, for example, might immediately start using rotator cuff therapy. That could make the problem worse, not better.

Ruppert has a background that has given her exceptional insight into the best way to help breast cancer patients conquer restricted range of motion caused by surgery. Her background is in spinal cord injuries.

> Patients with spinal cord injuries often present to rehab with shoulder dysfunction related to kyphotic [rounded] posture and poor body mechanics from wheelchair use. Treatment approaches for these patients include postural correction, myofascial release, scapular stabilization, upper extremity range of motion and strengthening. Chest wall scar tissue formation from surgical intervention and radiation therapy can lead to similar postural and body mechanic abnormalities. Given these similarities, it is presumed that we can use similar techniques to promote scapular retraction, upright posture and improved shoulder positioning. Once the shoulder sits in its neutral position, range of motion and strength can be addressed.[25]

Ruppert was correct. So when range-of-motion challenges result from scar tissue forming in the chest wall, a therapist has to use a hands-on technique to break up the scar tissue or work the connective tissue; the latter is called myofascial release. That helps to promote a more normal posture. From there, the patient can begin doing exercises to address the range of motion.

It's important for women to start rehab right after their initial surgery. Keeping the scar tissue that's forming as thin and flexible as possible makes recovery of function much easier. Even though they may not feel like coming to rehab after such a radical procedure, it's the best way to keep posture and range of motion as close to baseline as possible—baseline meaning the motion they had just before surgery rather than what they had when they were in high school. It also puts them in an improved position for their reconstruction, which may be months down the road. Reconstruction surgery can cause scarring, too, of course, so the patient isn't finished with rehab when she gets her new breasts.

In doing her initial assessment, Ruppert wants to know what sensations the patient has, too. Surgery involving the chest wall can easily cause nerve injury, both in the skin and the front part of the chest. One of two things might happen: either increased sensation or decreased sensation. So the patient might have chronic discomfort or pain, or she might have numbness in the area. If there is hypersensitivity, any touch to the area might be uncomfortable—and that might persist for quite a while. A woman who might have thought of her breasts as an erogenous zone and loved to have them touched might find that kind of touch impossible to tolerate until the nerves heal.

In the meantime, there is a fix for that, and women might even take pleasure in the process. In helping to promote tolerance to different levels of touch, a therapist might teach the patient how and when to apply a topical anesthetic like lidocaine. Many people are familiar with this numbing agent because they've used a lidocaine product to counter the pain of a bad sunburn. The use of a topical anesthetic can help the patient to retrain the areas to accept touch, whether it's the touch of a car seatbelt, a bra, or a partner's hand. The arousing part of the therapy is potentially the application of the lidocaine as part of foreplay.

Anecdotally, patients have not reported that nipple-sparing surgery does anything to preserve the kind of sensations that make some women's breasts an erogenous zone. It's a surgical technique that may enhance appearance, but it doesn't seem to have a bearing on function.

NONMEDICAL ESSENTIALS

Although there is a health-related reason why some of the guidance in this section is necessary, none of these suggestions is medical in nature. They are practical tips we've collected from women, primarily from gynecologic oncology patients as well as women who have gone through breast cancer.

At the top of the list is a relatively new product—approved for use in the United States in 2015, but in use in Europe since the 1970s—that can prevent one of the most profoundly awful effects of chemotherapy: hair loss. The *cold cap* looks a little like a bicycle helmet and serves to cool the scalp during a chemo treatment. The cap reduces blood flow to the scalp, so it minimizes the amount of medication that reaches it. Patients have reported absolute delight with the result; for many women, losing their hair is the ultimate insult and the one side effect that would most undermine their self-perception of being desirable.

A cold cap is tight fitting and filled with a gel that's extremely cold (−15 to −40 degrees Fahrenheit) to shrink the blood vessels in the scalp. The protocol for wearing the caps is somewhere between twenty and fifty minutes before, during, and after, but the protocol changes depending on what type of chemo you are receiving.

There is a tiny downside to the cold cap: You can't blow dry your hair, use hot rollers or straightening irons, or dye your hair during this process and for a few weeks that follow. What woman wouldn't choose the cold cap and those limitations over baldness? The larger downside is the expense. Until insurers are pressed to understand the mental health and emotional value of the device, they will continue to pull back from covering the cost. As of this writing, the company that makes the only cold cap approved for use in the United States is negotiating with insurance companies to get coverage for patient use.

The rest of the guidance has broader applicability to women who have gone through the cancer experience, but the emphasis remains on the types of problems and solutions to those problems that apply directly to women who have gone through cancer.

- Use a generous amount of lubricating jelly (aka gel) during intercourse. You do not want something that's watery or sticky, but rather something that provides relatively long-lasting glide. Generally, we would steer you toward water-based, water-soluble, odorless, and nonstaining lubricants. One reason is that the lubricant used to prevent stenosis during brachytherapy treatments must be water based. There is a silicon-formula alternative, however, that a number of patients have praised, and it can be used after brachy treatments are over. The silicon formula is water resistant so it gives you a little more flexibility in terms of the environment where intercourse occurs.
- On an ongoing basis, use pure, unfiltered coconut oil as a vaginal conditioner. Some therapists also recommend Vitamin E oil, although it tends to be a bit messier to use. Either one contributes to skin integrity, keeping the vagina soft, although they have limited value as a lubricant for sexual intercourse.
- Stay well hydrated. Your body has been through a lot no matter what cancer treatments you've experienced. It is very important to keep cleansing it from within by drinking water and other drinks designed to aid your electrolyte balance. There are pharmaceutical-grade hydration products available over the counter in powder form. In the United States, "pharmaceutical grade" means the product meets purity and absorption standards and that manufacturing occurred in certain facilities registered with the U.S. Food and Drug Administration (FDA).

- Wear whatever clothes you need, or turn up the thermostat, to be sure you are warm enough during sex. Some patients expressed concern that their exotic lingerie left them cold and uncomfortable, particularly while they were still going through chemotherapy. It could be time to invest in socks that match your lingerie. Gert Holstege, MD, PhD, chairman of the center for uroneurology at the University of Groningen in the Netherlands, conducted a 2005 study in which he found that the number of female subjects who were able to achieve orgasm in his study rose from 50 percent to 80 percent when he gave them socks. He has a research-based explanation: "In order to calm the amygdala and prefrontal cortex—the brain areas responsible for anxiety, fear, and danger signals—you need to be in a pleasant environment in which you feel safe, secure, and comfortable."[26] So, to refer back to a point made earlier in this chapter: You would do well to hold your partner's hand and then put your socks on.
- Now that we've discussed the value of socks, a decidedly unsexy component of your wardrobe, take a tip from Allis about underwear. Recall from chapter 5 that Allis had a pelvic exenteration and ended up with no vagina and two bags on her abdomen. She felt her confidence skyrocket when she created an alluring bedroom ensemble that hid the parts of her body that made her feel undesirable. The investment is in your self-esteem, and the level of your self-esteem feeds directly into your desire to connect intimately.
- Use exercise to boost your energy and strength while you reduce your stress. Do it every week of your life from now on and your sex life will improve. You don't have to make a commitment to work out that consumes huge amounts of time; just twenty minutes a day for five or six days a week is going to make a big difference in raising your level of endorphins. Like sex, exercise is "good stress" that stimulates the production of these neurochemicals that are structurally similar to morphine. They perform similarly in countering pain while they make you feel good. Part of the body's natural "reward" or "feel-good" system, the production of endorphins is stimulated by motherhood and eating a good meal as well as exercise and sexual activity. This all goes back to the discussion above about compassion for yourself; that is, addressing your needs and wants first so that you can be a good partner. An unsurprising corollary to the endorphin argument for exercise comes from a study done by Brooks, which makes running shoes and apparel. They concluded that 41 percent of women and 59 percent of men feel sexually stimulated after jogging.[27]

- Invest in sex toys. A good vibrator doesn't have to be expensive, but it does need to have a few different settings to suit your mood and desires at any given moment. It is the sex toy that *nearly every woman we interviewed* found essential. The reason is that its use can almost invariably lead to clitoral orgasm. But sex toys have another value, and women who have experienced sexual dysfunction and/or are older should explore that value: finding the G-spot. The G-spot, named for German gynecologist Ernst Gräfenberg, is an erogenous area at the upper part of the vagina. It's not uncommon for a young woman with a new lover to have the G-spot stimulated during intercourse and have an explosive orgasm. It's less common for an older woman who has a long-time partner to experience the same pleasure. But it isn't impossible. With a combination of pelvic floor exercises, such as the Kegels referenced above, and self-exploration with the appropriate sex toy, you can very likely find that spot and share the good news with your partner.

· 8 ·

Your New Normal

In all cases, we will explore ways for her to be intimate with her partner—even if traditional intercourse isn't possible given her new anatomy. Oftentimes, I am telling patients about their "new normal." Each couple has to establish what their new normal is.

—Lisa M. Ruppert, MD
Memorial Sloan Kettering Cancer Center

You want to press the reset button on life—both sexually and emotionally. The new normal is an opportunity.

—Jenni Skyler, PhD, LMFT, CST

Chapter 5 featured the story of Allis, who survived because she had the most extensive pelvic surgery possible. She and Craig now have a fulfilling life of sexual intimacy for reasons that can be analyzed, understood, and applied in other relationships. Chapter 4 hints at how they orchestrated their success; that is, they reduced their stress and learned to engage their parasympathetic nervous system by adding predictability and control to their sex life. They plan for sex; they know how to achieve mutual satisfaction.

This chapter is designed to help you bring home the lessons of such stories and to apply the solutions expressed throughout the book. It includes questions that help you and your partner reflect on what you have already read and figure out things, such as: "We're here, not there" "I'm this, not that."

In this chapter, we aim to help you bring together your understanding of the impact of cancer on intimate relationships and options for overcoming sexual functioning problems. As a result, we hope you will be equipped to use the guidance in the book to help design a future with sexual and marital pleasure.

A SURPRISE ABOUT MEN

An endometrial cancer patient in for a follow-up appointment complained harshly about her husband to her doctor, who contributed this story to us.

The doctor recalled her using a blistering tone and repeating, "He doesn't care. He just doesn't care." The interesting twist is that the husband was in the room at the time. He looked forlorn when he heard her accusations. In desperation, he finally said, "I don't know what to do. I massage her feet. I don't make her do work. I tried to support her in every way while she was getting chemo. All she does is lash out at me."

Her doctor could see this wasn't going in a good direction.

Suddenly, she started to cry. "I'm gonna die!"

"Why do you think you're going to die?" the doctor asked. She had finished her treatments months before that and showed no signs of a recurrence. She kept sobbing, so he finally said, "You need to live your life. And you need to keep in mind that no human being deserves to be a Dammit Doll." Dammit Dolls are durable fabric dolls designed to help someone relieve stress by "choking" it, slamming it on a table, stomping on it, or otherwise abusing it. We've all been guilty of treating another person like a Dammit Doll, but there is a big difference between slipping into that kind of offensive behavior occasionally and regularly targeting a loved one.

Hearing her doctor—the authority figure in the white coat who had performed life-saving surgery—speak with that kind of directness made her back off. It shocked her into paying attention. "Go on," she told him.

"Men tend to need physical and overt signs of affection even more than women do," he said. This began a conversation that opened the patient's eyes to how self-focused she had been. She had shut out the possibility of pleasure with her husband because she hadn't made herself available to connection with him on any level. He massaged her feet almost daily, and she wouldn't even hold his hand occasionally.

The doctor in this scenario was not just saying something to wake the patient up. His statement was based on some surprising research published in 2011 by the Kinsey Institute for Research in Sex, Gender, and Reproduction. Despite the long-held assumption that women need to be kissed, cuddled, and caressed more than men, the opposite turned out to be true—at least for couples who have been together for a while. The study that involved one thousand couples from the United States, Brazil, Germany, Spain, and Japan documented that these displays of affection are more important to men than they are to women. All of the couples were in committed relationships, with twenty-five years being average length of time they had been together.

The Kinsey study also held very good news for women in a long-term relationship—an insight that women trying to regain sexual functioning should plant in their head:

Men did report more relationship happiness in later years, whereas for women, their sexual satisfaction increased over time. Women who had been with their partner for less than 15 years were less likely to report sexual satisfaction, but after 15 years, the percentage went up significantly.[1]

A SURPRISE ABOUT WOMEN

"Sexual Activity in Midlife Women" is a multiyear study that was published by *JAMA* (*Journal of the American Medical Association*) *Internal Medicine* in 2014. It began in 2005, when 602 women first completed the Female Sexual Function Index (FSFI), the same short questionnaire that was included in the University of Colorado study. Study participants were in various stages of menopause and ranged in age from forty to sixty-five. They were screened for medical conditions, so it's appropriate to say that this was a healthy population at baseline.

Four years later, the team of researchers from the Center for Research on Healthcare at the University of Pittsburgh reconnected with the women and asked them to update the information on their level of sexual activity. At the time, 354 of the women indicated that they were sexually active, with 68 having missing data, which brought the study group down to 534. That translates to a total of 66.3 percent of women still being sexually active.

Year eight was even more revealing, with 85.4 percent of the women saying they were still sexually active. Specifically, they answered "yes" to the question: "During the past 6 months, have you engaged in *any* sexual activities with a partner?"[2] (Emphasis on *any* in the question was in the survey.) At that point, the study population ranged from forty-eight to seventy-three years of age. There is no indication how many of the women who stopped being sexually active had an illness, but it's highly likely some of them did.

The researchers reported two newsworthy conclusions:

1. "These findings challenge prior assumptions about female sexual function in midlife."[3]
2. In their opinion, the numbers were lower than if they had used a different instrument. (This is one reason why the University of Colorado study was far more robust; it used the nineteen questions of the FSFI, but incorporated far more questions about the quality of intimacy.)

What we can draw from this is what we said up front: Cancer and its treatments have a huge impact on sexual function—and that's to be expected. Without the cancer experience, these same women who participated in the UC sexual dysfunction study might be right up there with healthy subjects in the Pittsburgh study.

What we've seen is that some of them, one by one, are rejoining that population of sexually active women in midlife. They have decided to try to regain sexual intimacy after they are declared cured, have confidence in their remission, or simply commit to having a dynamic love life regardless of their chances of long-time survival.

WHERE WERE YOU?

Your baseline in terms of sexual functioning isn't how you felt when you were three months from graduating from college. It isn't where you were sexually when your sweetheart put thirty candles on your cake. Your baseline is how you experienced sex, what felt good, and who you were psychologically and physically just before you had surgery for cancer.

Consider this story from Lisa Ruppert, MD, at Memorial Sloan Kettering Cancer Center as you determine "where you were" prior to cancer.

> I had one patient who admitted she was chronically constipated as a child and her mother had to give her suppositories. She always struggled [with voiding] and she leaked throughout her life. As an adult, everyone told her she had weak muscles, so she did Kegels. She told me, "It never actually helped."
>
> She had surgery for a gyn cancer and had scarring in that area. She noticed she was struggling even more with her bowel and her bladder. Interestingly enough, she was someone who was hypertonic in the pelvic floor muscles and never knew how to relax. A lot of women struggle with that because they harbor their stress in their pelvic floor. It's that notion, "I just went to the bathroom. I'm really stressed. I have to go again." She was like that. Then you give her scar tissue and she was even tighter and struggling even more.
>
> All of her therapy was just geared toward teaching her to relax. After therapy, she was more continent than she had ever been in her entire life. No one ever told her that the problem was not that she wasn't contracting her muscles; it's that she wasn't relaxing them.
>
> Cancer is an unfortunate diagnosis, but sometimes the experience you have on the backside does change things for you for the better. Some patients do come back to say and say, "I'm better now than before I was diagnosed."[4]

If there was one surprise that rose to the top after a number of interviews, it was this: Where a couple was in terms of intimacy prior to a cancer diagnosis was often *below* the level of intimacy they achieved going through cancer together.

We don't want to mislead you on this. In some cases, they had very goal-oriented (translate: orgasm focused) sexual intercourse, and they described it in terms such as *great* and *amazing*. Afterward, some of them couldn't even have intercourse, or at least not have it very often. But the satisfaction they got in their sexual relationship—though not the same as precancer—was better in many cases. By "better" they mean it was more varied and, by the woman's standards, more fulfilling.

WHERE ARE YOU NOW?

Right now, regardless of what phase of the cancer experience you are in, how would you describe your sexual functioning? Choose as many options as applicable.

   a. Normal disruption. Considering what we're gone through (or are still going through), this was to be expected.
   b. Definite impact on psychological/emotional ability to connect intimately. Issues are things such as self-esteem, fears, anger, sadness, defeat . . .
   c. Definite impact on physical ability to connect intimately. Issues are things such as pain, dryness, constriction of vagina, loss of muscle tone . . .
   d. We didn't have sex much (or at all) before this disease showed up, so loss of sexual functioning doesn't mean much.

Let's address the last one first. If you chose d, then why did you buy or borrow this book? You're here, having made it all the way to chapter 8, because you have some interest in regaining sexual function. Keep reading.

NORMAL DISRUPTION

Before surgery, chemotherapy, or radiation, a nurse hands you a packet or a three-ring binder with instructions, side effects, self-care tips, support resources, and much more. You go into treatment experiences, therefore, with your health care team having managed your expectations about "normal disruptions" and how to address them. In a way, that's as bizarre as someone giving you a book on raising a teenage girl and saying, "Here's everything you need to know!"

Like raising a teenage girl, experiencing cancer and its treatments is full of surprises. "Normal disruption" is relative, as in, what do you consider "normal"?

That said, it is possible to go from diagnosis through treatment and feel as though your journey followed a course that was, for the most part, predictable. You could warn your partner about your hair possibly growing in kinky, or that you would require extreme gentleness in your attempts to make love. There were still surprises—every person is different—but there were no shocks.

If that's how you would describe your experience, and yet you would put yourself in the category of someone having some measure of sexual dysfunction, then we hope you explore the stories about solutions and descriptions of solutions in this book. You can both consider yourself and your relationship and your journey "normal" or "typical" and still have snags in your sex life.

To give you another perspective on what is normal or typical, we conducted a nonscientific survey. The results gave us some very predictable results, as well as some good news about what may be considered typical—at least in the United States—in relation to the cancer experience.

On September 13, 2016, one hundred residents in the United States responded to a ten-question survey about "people they were close to" who had experienced either gynecologic or breast cancer. The respondent was also invited to answer if she had gone through either category of cancer herself, but this survey did not ask the individual to divulge that. Here are the characteristics of the group:

52 percent female
48 percent male

Age:
18–29   21 percent
30–44   26 percent
45–60   28 percent
> 60   25 percent

Residing in thirty-two different states in the continental United States.

The results were as follows:

- Twenty-seven percent were close to someone who had gone through a gynecologic cancer (or had gone through it herself)
- Fifty-one percent were close to someone who had gone through breast cancer (or had gone through it herself)

It wasn't possible to ascertain how much overlap there was between the two groups because of the structure of the survey. That is, we were not sure how many people were close to a woman who'd had gynecologic cancer as well as a woman who'd had breast cancer. Realizing that we weren't doing the survey with a "scientific method" in mind—we were just looking for a rough idea of the experiences of a random one hundred people—we then calculated percentages on the basis of the larger number, 51 percent. In other words, if forty-five people said they were close to someone who'd had cancer and she had been in great pain after treatment, then that would mean forty-five of fifty-one people, or 88 percent, saw their friend or relative experiencing a lot of pain. With that numerical relationship in mind,

- Eighty-eight percent of those who were close to someone who'd had one of these cancers said that the woman experienced a lot of pain as a result of treatment.
- Eighty-four percent said the woman had lost her hair because of treatment.
- Fourteen percent said she separated from her partner or spouse within three years of the diagnosis (In the UC study, 10 percent of all women reported separating from their partner for some time. Note: This was not a number that the study considered statistically significant).
- Six percent saw that person get a divorce within three years. (In the UC study, 5 percent of all women reported separating from their partner. Note: This was not a number that the study considered statistically significant).
- Sixty-nine percent said that the woman expressed feelings of looking unattractive during treatment.

After that, we added three questions seeking "good news." These numbers are uplifting because they were total unknowns, unlike the five above that addressed pain, hair loss, relationship issues, and feelings of undesirability.

- Thirty percent indicated that the woman stated that her experience of cancer helped her relationship with her partner or spouse.

- Fifty-seven percent said that the woman admitted that cancer helped her be a better person; for example, more resilient or more patient.
- Seventy-five percent said that the woman took action to help other cancer patients get through the experience, such as volunteering with Relay for Life, writing a blog, or helping with a support group.

What we would therefore offer you as a takeaway from this subsection on "normal disruption" is that there are predictable short-term physical effects that will undermine sexual functioning. In some cases, they also affect self-image. In a small number of cases, they seem to lead to relationship dysfunction. But look at the other "typical" numbers! A healthy chunk of people saw cancer as a path to improving relationships as well as self-improvement and a strengthened connection to community.

Jeff, the husband of one of the UC study participants, was quite insightful in describing the normal disruption he and his wife experienced, as well as how they dealt with it. He first targeted greater-than-usual discrepancy in desire as part of what he and his wife experienced during and right after her cancer treatments. Jenni Skyler, PhD, founder of the Intimacy Institute, reinforces the notion that such a discrepancy is not only common, it's also normal: "Unless it's the honeymoon period, there's nearly always a discrepancy. The biggest reason that couples come to therapy is that it becomes significant."[5]

Jeff shared some important insights about recovering from that kind of normal disruption and discovering renewed intimacy:

> To me, the most important component is that the woman *wants* to have sex. Part of supporting her recovery from cancer is supporting her efforts to regain a sense of being a desirable sex partner. After my wife lost her hair, we went to the American Cancer Society together and she tried on wigs. We had fun—she looked very sassy as a redhead—but we also teared up when she found the right one. She looked normal. It was her birthday, so I took my strawberry blonde date to a celebratory lunch.
>
> The physical limitations right after treatment are insignificant compared to the mental ones. As soon as my wife felt ready, I felt desired by her and I desired her—hair or no hair, scars or no scars.
>
> When a woman feels a vibrant sex life is behind her, it doesn't matter what her partner does to bring it forward. She has to see it as a current reality. And what we discovered is that the reality had more variations for us after cancer than it had since we'd started dating decades before that. We road-tested different lubes, brought a vibrator into the act, and decided that any room in the house was suitable. We also took a few short trips together. Spending the night in a different location can rev up interest in being together sexually.

My goal was never to re-create what we had before my wife had the procedures, but to have a pleasant, healthy sex life in the here and now. We aim to be playful and to explore options that we didn't consider previously.

A healthy sex life is mostly mental. The physical aspects of sex are pretty straightforward. They haven't varied much since we lost our virginity. I don't mean to minimize the physical part of this—cancer can have a big, negative impact on that—but it's how you think about it, how creative you can be together, that helps restore the passion.

PSYCHOLOGICAL/EMOTIONAL IMPACT

The truth? We didn't interview a single woman or man affected by gynecologic or breast cancer who escaped having this disease impact their psychological/emotional ability to connect intimately. Regardless of how "normal" they perceived the disruptions to be—or how they maintained great emotional strength in face of constipation, cystitis, depression, hair loss, vomiting, and pain—they felt a profound psychological/emotional blow to their intimate relationship.

Jenni Skyler has a thriving clinical practice in sex therapy and gives entertaining "sex talks" in the Boulder, Colorado, area. Her success rate may relate to the fact that, like author Mary Roach (*Bonk*), she's very funny when she talks about sex—and that puts people at ease.

The foundation of Skyler's approach to helping clients is to be educational while she gives people permission for healthy and pleasurable conversations about human sexuality. The humor is invitational, geared to the demographics of her audience. For clients going through a cancer experience to regain sexual intimacy, her approach has three parts:

1. *Reframe your experience as an opportunity.* This is a chance to get to know your own sexuality like never before.

Other couples may not have gone through such a big bump in the road, but you have felt the shudder of the bump and now you are moving on.

We sometimes fall into a pattern of taking each other for granted. We fall into a loveless and sexless relationship, or lower love and lower sex. We are on autopilot going through the motions of life and then we hit this big bump in the road and it makes us hypersensitive to everything that's supposedly "going wrong."

We have to find ourselves and each other again.

2. *Survivors of cancer and the caregiver/partner have to know: We are all students of our own sexuality.* And we are students of each other's sexuality—lifelong students.

After cancer treatment, we need to learn the newness of a partner's body, the way we love to be touched, our human sexual response, and the new way our nerve endings respond to touch. Especially after having chemo and radiation, nerve endings feel different and react differently—at least for awhile. Orgasm may be a whole different experience, and sometimes, it can be elusive.

How we learn to interact with one another, how we learn to turn on each other's brains and bodies, may be quite different from what we had before. Sometimes, as in the case of Allis and Craig, intercourse is completely off the table. For other couples, it may be the alternate form of pleasure rather than the main event.

For any cancer that a woman survives, the vagina can take a big hit. The vaginal tissue may become very thin with the potential of tearing easily. Hormone therapy is not an option for some because it could increase the risk of another cancer. The message is therefore to open your mind about sex. What is it? What do you want out of it? What will give your partner pleasure?

3. *Redefine sex.* What is sex? In chapter 2, we talked about how sex works in a medical sense, but that is different from defining sex in the context of a long-term, intimate relationship. Sklyer says about the "medical" characterization of sex:

> Let's ditch that modality of thinking of and having sex in a performance oriented way and let's just have a Cheesecake of Pleasure. We want to redefine sex as a more holistic and comprehensive understanding of sensual contact.
>
> When we change our minds about the definition of sex, we change how we behave as intimate beings with each other.
>
> When you think your partner might die—even if it's a fleeting thought—it's normal to hold back from letting yourself be vulnerable. It's not usually a conscious decision, but a subconscious reaction to hold back from connection for fear of losing the other person. You can look at it from both sides. If you're the cancer patient, you can say to yourself, "If I pull back from connection and get really sick and die, it's better that I wasn't that connected to my partner." From the partner's perspective, it's "If I can disconnect, then I won't be as hurt if/when she dies."
>
> I've seen both the cancer patient and the caregiver hold back in certain areas because they are afraid of dropping deeply into love and then losing that partner.
>
> Upfront, we need to put that reality of grief on the table—grieving the reality that we are mortal beings. We all have a deadline at some point, but it doesn't preclude us from falling more deeply into intimacy, to be in the here and now and love each other. And to know that, yes, at the end of the day, one of us will go and that will be painful. But as the poet Alfred Lord Tennyson said, "Tis better to have loved and lost than never to have loved at all."[6]

Skyler noted that the cliché may be overworked, but it is one that couples going through cancer should look at with fresh perspective. In trying to reignite intimacy that was nearly extinguished by fear, it's important to remember how intrinsic love is to our sense of feeling alive.

Some couples who come to Skyler for insights on their sex lives cross the threshold into greater intimacy after a single visit. They quickly get the image she gives them of typical sex being like a staircase—or to use another cliché, it's the "Stairway to Heaven" (thank you, Led Zeppelin). In other words, in that initial session, they have the a-ha moment that sex isn't about performance. They understand that sex isn't a succession of predicted events that lead to a predicted outcome:

The Performance-Oriented Stairway to Heaven: Only one of many options!

END HERE: Have an orgasm

Have intercourse

Have genital contact

Take our clothes off

Kiss

START HERE: Get together

That's how Hollywood does it, and it's usually in about ninety seconds. This is the image that causes lingering anxiety with couples—even smart couples who are deeply in love—because the image is extremely difficult to abandon. It's a performance-oriented, goal-oriented model of sex that makes it less fun. Trash that.

The alternative that Skyler talks about is the Cheesecake of Pleasure, wherein you see sexual intimacy as a source of pleasure but orgasm is not the goal. Your journey is a tasting experience, with each sexual activity delivering a different kind of pleasure. And you can have whatever piece you want.

Here is how it might look:

1. Prepare to share the cheesecake by having a solo date. Know your own body so you know what you're sharing with your partner.
2. Know what turns you on mentally. Get to know the literature and film that ignites your sexual fantasies.
3. Engage in sensual massage.
4. Engage in sensual massage involving the genitals.
5. Have a kissing date. Everything you do is kissing from head to toe.
6. Caress the genitals with your hands.
7. Caress the genitals with your mouth.

8. Cook together. Enjoying the many textures and flavors of food can be erotic.
9. Play with the genitals. A little vibration, a smooth move . . .
10. Indulge in intercourse using a lot of lube.
11. Indulge in intercourse with various positions.
12. Find exotic places to have sex, whether or not it's intercourse, like the car or in the bedroom at your mother's house.
13. Have fun with lube. There are so many different kinds, and each can promote pleasure in a unique way.
14. Have fun with toys. See the above note on the advantages of different lubes.

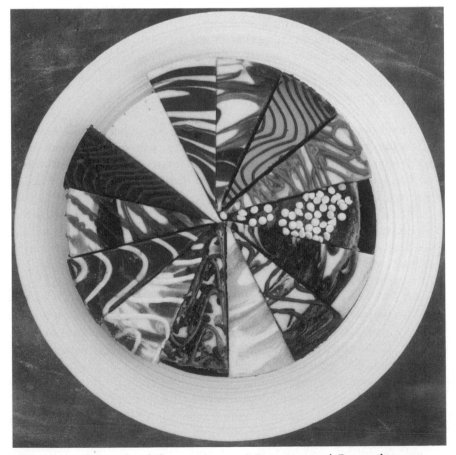

Figure 8.1.   Cheesecake of Pleasure. *Source:* © Peanutroaster | Dreamstime.com

Skyler guides her clients in the "flavors of pleasure" by saying:

This can be framed and understood as 15 minutes per slice of cheesecake. Take that time, or whatever time you need or want, to indulge in a sensual activity, purely for the sake of pleasure. Pleasure is the goal! Couples must agree on all slices included in the cheesecake. Slices can be very vanilla or very full of fruits, nuts, and chocolate. My only rule is enthusiastic consent. Example flavors can be sensual massage, sensual showers, mutual masturbation, intercourse, manual stimulation, oral sex, anal sex, play with dildos, play with vibrators, play with blindfolds, and on and on.

Jenni Skyler's Cheesecake of Pleasure is all about your mind. You have probably been told since you first learned about sex that what you want is an orgasm, and what your partner wants is an orgasm. What you want is pleasure. And that's what your partner wants as well—amazing, mind-blowing pleasure. The big surprise in learning about sexual intimacy is that pleasure comes in many different flavors.

As a bridge to the discussion of your new normal after feeling the physical impact of the cancer experience, we want to focus on female arousal disorder. The link between the psychological and physical is that this sexual dysfunction is construed as "in the mind," but one of the solutions is a drug.

Generalized hypoactive sexual desire disorder (HSDD) is characterized by low sexual desire and affects an estimated 10 percent of women, according to the International Society for Sexual Medicine. It is not partner specific, meaning that it's not a manifestation of problems in a relationship. Even if a woman's favorite movie star showed up for a tryst, she might not go beyond offering a cup of coffee. HSDD is a problem when it causes anxiety or depression about the state of the woman's main interpersonal relationship. Another characteristic of the disorder is that it is not caused by medication, so this might be something that a woman acquired long after she completed cancer treatments.

In August 2015, the U.S. Food and Drug Administration (FDA) approved Addyi (flibanserin) for use in treating HSDD in premenopausal women. As of this writing, it is the only FDA-approved treatment for the disorder. *Vogue* magazine's Amy Gamerman accurately captured the difference between Addyi and Viagra, which is a vasodilator used to treat erectile dysfunction:

Addyi [is] a peach-colored pill that offers women the possibility of eros regained. Its arrival marks the culmination of years of trial, development, and controversy. The first medication ever approved for female sexual dysfunction in premenopausal women, Addyi has been called the "pink Viagra." The label is erroneous. Viagra is a tool designed for a man's faulty hydraulics. Addyi aspires to the metaphysical, targeting a woman's brain chemistry in order to boost her desire.[7]

Metaphysical is a rather lofty word to describe the effects of Addyi, but the message is on target. That is, flibanserin works on serotonin receptors in the brain to improve libido. Serotonin is associated with mood balance; if your brain isn't getting enough, you might fall into depression.

The population that will likely benefit from Addyi is relatively small if you remove those for whom it's contraindicated. If you have low blood pressure or are committed to having that glass of wine with dinner every night, then Addyi is not for you. Drinking alcohol is prohibited when you take this drug. Here's another downer: You have to take it every day, and it takes more than a month for the effects to kick in.

But let's end this look at the pink pill on a high note by citing what the *Vogue* author, the mother of four and married to her husband for many years, concluded after taking Addyi for several weeks:

> I'm suddenly thinking more about sex. I am not obsessed, just newly alert to erotic possibility, scanning the world around me for any sign of it. I study my husband's body. *Not bad. Has he been working out?* I scrutinize each woman I pass on the street. *Does she still want it?* At yoga class I stretch on my mat and try to quiet my thoughts. The instructor places her hand on my back. *Her skin feels warm. . . . Do I smell bergamot?*[8]

It's estimated that the drug works only with about 20 to 30 percent of women who try it, but you don't know until you do if you are going to be one of the fortunate ones like the writer for *Vogue*.

PHYSICAL IMPACT

If you selected c above because you feel that there are physical barriers to establishing a new normal in your sexual intimacy, first ascertain if any of the following applies to you:

- Pain during intercourse
- Hypersensitivity to touch
- Numbness in erogenous areas
- Vaginal dryness
- Vaginal tightness
- Muscle weakness in the pelvic area

All of these problems, which tend to be relatively common after cancer treatments, were addressed specifically in chapter 7 in the medical and nonmedical discussions of solutions. You may not be able to solve the problem completely, but in most cases, you can reduce the impact on your sex life.

Now let's go further into a condition we touched on only briefly before: the inability to have an orgasm, or inorgasmia. We described the types of inorgasmia (known by many therapists as anorgasmia) in chapter 6, so now let's look at what you might do about it.

One of the most common causes is certain types of antidepressants. If the cancer experience left you feeling depressed, that may have prompted your family doctor to prescribe a selective serotonin reuptake inhibitor (SSRI). You would have lots of company going to the drug store since nearly one in five women in the United States takes an antidepressant, according to the Centers for Disease Control and Prevention.[9] You are also part of a crowd if the medicine caused your libido to plummet: Roughly 70 percent of women report reduced sexual desire while taking antidepressants.[10] FDA-approved SSRIs are

- Citalopram (Celexa)
- Escitalopram (Lexapro)
- Fluoxetine (Prozac)
- Paroxetine (Paxil, Pexeva)
- Sertraline (Zoloft)
- Vilazodone (Viibryd)
- Fluvoxamine, which is approved to treat obsessive-compulsive disorder but is sometimes used to treat depression

Since Addyi also affects serotonin levels, you might wonder why SSRIs turn down your libido while Addyi can turn it up. Pat yourself on the back: It's a superb research question also posed by numerous physicians as well as *Scientific American* in an article examining Addyi two months after FDA approval. The answer is that some physicians are prescribing it to treat depression—this is considered an off-label use—in the hope that patients will get the benefits of countering depression without undermining their sex life. This is one controversy that requires us to stay tuned to the latest research in order to give you more answers.

Medical problems that may have been exacerbated by the cancer experience, such as hypertension or diabetes, can also result in inorgasmia. It is important that you communicate the fact that you have a problem achieving orgasm to the physician treating you if you find it bothersome.

Finally, abuse is a big cause of inorgasmia. The source can be physical or psychological, but the result is physical. Cancer patients are not excluded from the large population of women who experience abuse, and it is wrong to assume that a spouse or partner will "go easy" on a woman against whom he has perpetrated some kind of violence just because she's sick. Even in this discussion, however, there is good news. Physicians such as gynecologists and gynecologic oncologists who specialize in women's health challenges not only receive special training to spot abuse but they also hone their instincts to identify women at risk. In general, members of their staff also have this kind of training.

There is no magic pill like Addyi to address inorgasmia, although studies involving women taking Viagra have yielded some interesting results. While Viagra wouldn't work for HSDD, there is some research to suggest that it can help with postmenopausal female sexual arousal disorder (FSAD). With this disorder, the women cannot achieve or maintain sexual excitement; hence, the inability to climax.

One study—and we should mention that it was funded by Viagra maker Pfizer, Inc.—pitted the drug against a placebo. The 202 women in the study either were postmenopausal or they had had a hysterectomy. The team conducting the study, documented in *The Journal of Urology*, focused on how the women answered two questions:

- After taking the study medication, the sensation/feeling in my genital (vagina, labia, clitoris) area during intercourse or stimulation seemed to be: (a) more than before, (b) less than before, or (c) unchanged.
- After taking the study medication, intercourse and/or foreplay was (a) pleasant and satisfying, better than before taking the study medication; (b) unpleasant, worse than before the study medication; (c) unchanged, no difference; or (d) pleasant but still not like it used to be or I would like it to be.[11]

After weeding out the study participants who had HSDD, the research team found that 69 percent of the women who took Viagra reported improvement in sensation in their genital area during intercourse or stimulation. They concluded, therefore, that the women who took Viagra were eight times more likely to report physical improvement than those who had the placebo.

So should you take Viagra if you have problems climaxing? No. At least, not yet. We don't have enough research on possible side effects, which could be dramatic, particularly if you're on other medications. As with Addyi, check to see what the latest research is and then discuss it with a physician who has actually read the latest research.

BURY ONE WORD; BIRTH ANOTHER

Dyspareunia. We have used this word once before in the first chapter and kept it out of our vocabulary ever since. It's the medical term for painful intercourse—and we know by now that "painful intercourse" can also mean the mental pain associated with any form of sexual intimacy.

By urging you to bury the word, we are not encouraging you to avoid the concept of sexual dysfunction. Instead, we hope to lure you away from medical labels of problems and lure you toward medical and nonmedical paths to opportunities for the "new normal" of your intimacy with another person.

If you do an online search on "dyspareunia antonym" as a way of finding the opposite of the "painful intercourse" word, you get "orgasm." A physician like Lisa Ruppert would probably tell you that's not medically correct, but here's how the thesaurus is correct: An orgasm is characterized by feelings of pleasure. In contrast, dyspareunia is characterized by displeasure, or some level of pain. In terms of sex therapy, then, it's easy to see how characterizing dyspareunia and orgasm as experiential opposites makes perfect sense.

Rabbi Shmuley Boteach, author of *Kosher Sex*, talks about the "tyranny of the visual"[12] that is pervasive in our society. It can keep people from being confident in sexual interactions with a partner. This is particularly true for couples who have experienced the cutting, catheters, and chemotherapy of cancer treatment. Boteach says,

> When you open your eyes during sex you achieve what I call "non-verbal communication." You begin to communicate in paragraphs, pages, whole chapters with a certain glance. And there's such an innocence, an honesty, a raw nakedness in that glance that can't be had in any other human interaction.
>
> . . . We've now discovered the power of things like pheromones—the scent of sex. And there's the sound of sex.
>
> The problem with sex in America is that everything is visual. Porn is a visual experience . . . and to an extent, I think we live under the tyranny of the visual where so many people feel uncomfortable about their body because they look at these "perfect" people and feel inadequate as a result. They cannot be sexually confident in their interaction with their spouse.
>
> What makes sex the most pleasurable of all human experiences is that you have the confidence to let go completely and submit to instinct. And the reason sex is so pleasurable is that it involves real liberation. It's one of the only times we human beings are free of inhibition. We're free of social constraints, and we submit entirely to what comes naturally. But if you can't submit because you have all these hang-ups, then sex becomes a hang-up experience and it's not pleasant and it's not pleasurable.[13]

What we've been driving toward in this book is the discovery or rediscovery of pleasure. So bury the bad word and start talking about your orgasms.

LET'S GO FOR IT

In *Bonk*, science author Mary Roach describes how arousal for someone with a spinal cord injury is sometimes quite unusual. She describes how areas of sensation—areas of sexual arousal—may not be at all associated with genitalia. We asked Memorial Sloan Kettering physiatrist Lisa Ruppert, whose approach to sexual dysfunction is grounded in her knowledge of spinal cord injuries, what was going on, and how did that knowledge apply to anyone and everyone who has experienced some kind of sexual dysfunction. She said,

> It's not that you develop new sensations. You become more aware. You can lose sensation in traditional areas.
>
> If you have a spinal cord injury, your motor or your sensory function is typically impaired below the spinal cord injury. But it's not always a complete thing. You don't necessarily lose "everything." You may retain things. Everyone is different.
>
> But what happens is that we have this social mindset that there are certain areas that you are going to touch for sexual arousal or intercourse and we adapt to them because that's what society tells us how we normally engage in sex. Well, those might be areas where you've lost sensation; *however*, you might have maintained sensation in other areas. And that might be sensation that is pleasurable to you, but it was never something that you explored before.
>
> So I encourage anyone who has sensory impairment: See what feels good. See where it feels good. Because you might actually find that, now you have areas that will stimulate you and excite you that are new to you. That's what we want to explore. Exploit those sites. Explore what really feels good to you.[14]

Explore on your own. Explore with your partner. Be honest. Tell your partner what feels good.

Conclusion:
Focus on the Partners

$\mathcal{O}$ne of the couples we interviewed is a married same-sex couple living in Manhattan. We had a hypothesis that a female partner would have the innate ability to be more empathetic about a gynecologic cancer than a male partner. We weren't proven wrong, but we weren't proven right, either. We mostly learned something about expectations of male and female behavior, and how those expectations can affect any couple going through cancer.

From many married men we interviewed, we heard that they wanted to be "the rock," "the source of strength." Two of them broke down in tears as they recalled what their wives went through. Several had to pause and take a breath before they could move forward with the interview. They were visibly and audibly trying to avert a crying episode. All of these men apologized.

For what? For having empathy?

The partner in the same-sex couple was "allowed" to be squeamish about the tubes coming out of her wife. No one questioned her tears or expected her to apologize for shedding them as she dug up memories of the drip line for chemo.

Igniting sexual intimacy during and after cancer has a lot to do with understanding what the partner has gone through, too. As hard as it is, if you're the one going through cancer, you need to look at that person who loves you and consider the levels of pain and doubt that have infected him or her as well. And it's critical to know how your behavior has affected that person's ability to function in a support role and to show affection to you.

Some patients become so discouraged by knowing they have cancer that they choose to give up. Those patients are tough to support; the expectation many people would have for that person's partner is, "Just show up."

We didn't interview anyone like that for this book. We interviewed patients who would share actor Michael Douglas's sentiment: "Cancer didn't bring me to my knees, it brought me to my feet." These are people who responded to concerned tears with "I love you, too!" and responded to displays of strength with "Thank you!" These are simple expressions of paying attention that open the door to intimacy.

In the throes of a cancer diagnosis and debilitating treatment, the patient's partner can sometimes make a huge difference with noncomplementary behavior. Vice versa: The patient can sometimes get the two of them on track with noncomplementary behavior.

Complementarity is the behavior we commonly have with another person, whether we know the person or not. You are pleasant to me, and I am pleasant to you. You grumble at me, I grumble at you.

Noncomplementarity runs counter to that. Mahatma Gandhi and Martin Luther King, Jr., famously returned hateful words with gentle ones, and violent actions with demonstrations of peace. There is no guarantee that such noncomplementary behavior will diffuse a situation, but the same ability to mirror another person gives us the ability to read a person's mood. If we carefully observe and listen, we can figure out if noncomplementary behavior is an appropriate strategy at the moment.

Here is how this might work. It had been twenty years since George had had a car accident, but he lost control and rear-ended a car driven by a middle-aged woman. She jumped out of the car screaming at him. The severity of her response far exceeded the damage to the cars and culminated in a personal attack: "Why would you do this to me?!" He listened as she told her story: This was her husband's car and they were getting a divorce. With kindness, he hugged her. This is an example of noncomplementary behavior.

In the case of a person who feels assaulted by disease and physically weak, other people might complement that behavior with sympathy and softness. They try to show support by taking their energy down a notch, to energetically be on the same plane as the other person. It's not necessarily a planned response, but an intuitive one. It's a complementary response that seems appropriate—a good way to make the patient not only feel comfortable but also feel more normal.

Sometimes, it may be effective. Other times, and some of this may depend on the person, a noncomplementary approach might be the best.

In other words, sometimes both patient and caregiver need to be aware that there is "stuff" going on, and getting sucked into it won't help. Sometimes, you have to look past the expression of emotion and try to see what the person really needs at the moment.

We want to close with inspiring words of gratitude from playwright Eve Ensler, a cancer survivor. Ensler was primarily known for her acclaimed play *The Vagina Monologues* until she put her own cancer in a book and onstage with *In the Body of the World: A Memoir of Cancer and Connection.* The metaphorical relationship she makes between her cancer and the diseases of the world embodies compelling images of human and environmental suffering. In the context of this book, however, a more important message is her description of what she learned by having and surviving cancer.

> What I learned is it has to do with attention and resources that everybody deserves. It was advocating friends and a doting sister. It was wise doctors and advanced medicine and surgeons who knew what to do with their hands. It was underpaid and really loving nurses. It was magic healers and aromatic oils. It was people who came with spells and rituals. It was having a vision of the future and something to fight for, because I know this struggle isn't my own. It was a million prayers. It was a thousand hallelujahs and a million oms. It was a lot of anger, insane humor, a lot of attention, outrage. It was energy, love and joy. It was all these things.[1]

Each of us who has experienced cancer will increase our capacity to enjoy greater intimacy and connection if we always remember to show gratitude to those who participated in our victory.

Appendix A:
Tips from Former Patients

Former and current cancer patients grouped their insights into Patient-to-Patient and Patient-to-Physician/Nurse tips. We included some of them in chapter 7 in the nonmedical solutions discussion, but a few didn't fit. These are a couple of Patient-to-Patient tips that could contribute to your ability to enjoy intimacy because they can greatly relieve your stress and/or allow you to channel anxiety to people other than your partner. And the Patient-to-Physician/Nurse tips we chose are those that suggest how to minimize fear; therefore, they will help couples feel as well informed and in control as possible during the cancer experience. Again, the point is to reduce stress, which tends to undermine sexual functioning as much, or more so, than the treatments themselves.

PATIENT-TO-PATIENT TIPS

Have an advocate. You may think that having a partner with you is all you need—and maybe that's true. The reality for many cancer patients, however, is that your partner is so emotionally engaged in the process that he or she is too distracted and distraught to focus concurrently on the details of your care, your schedule, your medications, and your bills.

Your advocate could be a professional, such as a member of the Alliance of Professional Health Advocates, or it could be a friend or relative. Professionals generally have experience navigating the system, asking good questions, exploring options, analyzing bills, working with insurance companies, and in some cases, they can even do lifestyle and fitness coaching. A friend or relative may do a great job, depending on your level of need. This is probably the case if you just need someone to help coordinate your care, remind you what questions to ask, and put another pair of eyes on your bill. The latter function is critical because the last thing a cancer patient needs is the burden of looking at a column of numbers (that is, amounts due) next to a list like this: lab services, chemistry, hematology, chest X-ray, clinic visit, pharmacy, IV therapy, chemotherapy, CT thorax w/contrast. Consider the additional stress a couple faces if one or both of them has to figure out what has been billed twice, why the explanation of benefits doesn't match the rest of the bill, and what procedure you were billed for that you didn't even have.

Have a support person/attend a support group. This is someone (or a group) who has gone through the type of cancer you are experiencing or is going through it.

Jeanene Smith is associate director of the Colorado Ovarian Cancer Alliance, which provides support to people affected by ovarian cancer in addition to promoting awareness and early detection of the disease. COCA has six support groups with monthly meetings that are all professionally led. Outside of those monthly meetings, some women might choose to get together to address deep emotional, family, and sexual issues. There is also a one-on-one mentoring program where concerns about intimacy could be addressed.

One of the former patients we interviewed described the value of her support group:

> I found myself wanting to connect with people who knew what this journey looked like. Having cancer can be very isolating. In the support group, I found a sisterhood that enabled me to learn from other women about managing the side effects of treatment, complementary treatment options, and that support helped to lift me out of my current experience and gave me hope. They helped me step through the process. The other women gave me tips and information that made it an easier journey.

Support groups give participants some immediate, meaningful feedback to their big concerns and big victories. It means women who feel joyful when they hear your CA 125 test result was 8. It means women who know what it feels like to have a husband look at them with concern when they want to see desire in his eyes.

Smith summarized the type of women who tend to participate in these groups in these words:

> The women who come to the groups tend to be very aware, self-educated women who can discuss treatment options and clinical trials. They are great self-advocates. These women are looking for answers and want to share those answers with other women. We've had women tell us anecdotally that they feel the information they learned from the support group is responsible for them still being alive.[1]

Unlike a physician or nurse who has never had the cancer experience you have had, you would find women who have personally addressed problems that are getting in the way of your sexual intimacy. You could take this book into the group and ask, "Have you tried this?"

PATIENT-TO-PHYSICIAN/NURSE TIPS

Help the patient ask you questions. Both the patient and her partner may not be aware that the doctor and nurse can answer questions about things such as sexual dysfunction. A simple question like "Is it normal to have incontinence after this surgery?" could lead to a vital referral to a pelvic floor rehabilitation specialist. To elicit that, it may be necessary to go beyond "Are you having any problems?" Go to the heart of the matter: "Are you having any problems with leaking urine, skin rashes, dry vagina . . . ?" Even the couple we spoke with who are both physicians felt that they didn't ask all of the questions they could have to avert certain problems during recovery.

Be honest about your limitations. Although we recounted two instances in which the physician "gave up" because the patient's needs seemed to exceed the doctor's ability, it's better than the opposite. The last thing a patient needs is a doctor admitting after the fact—as Allis's first surgeon did—that there were upsetting surprises during the surgery.

Have the right person make the phone call. One of the most upsetting things we heard in the interviews was recounted in chapter 5. Allis got a call from the nurse at her doctor's office, who told her she needed a CA 125 test. When Allis asked her what that was, the nurse replied, "It's not something I can discuss with you. I'll ask the doctor to call you." Bad form. The person who has the information the patient needs is the one who should make the call. That is an effective way to help a patient feel more centered and in control.

Appendix B:
Selected Resources Related to Intimacy and Cancer

Alliance of Professional Health Advocates (APHA) (www.aphadvocates.org)—A directory of private, professional, independent patient advocates and care professionals; getting an advocate involved can greatly reduce your stress.

American Association of Sexuality Educators, Counselors and Therapists (AASECT) (www.aasect.org)—Includes a range of professionals who share an interest in promoting understanding of human sexuality and healthy sexual behavior; facilitates locating someone near you.

American Cancer Society (ACS) (www.cancer.org)—Click on the tab "Find Support & Treatment" to get insights on coping with side effects, among other things; the same section provides insights on "Cancer, sex, and sexuality."

American Physical Therapy Association (APTA) (www.apta.org)—Members include physical therapists, physical therapist assistants, and students of physical therapy and will help you locate a qualified pelvic floor specialist near you.

Foundation for Women's Cancer (www.foundationforwomenscancer.org)—Sponsors courses throughout the country that include topics such as "Sexuality after Cancer" and provide educational videos online.

GoodTherapy.org (www.goodtherapy.org)—While the general focus is on a range of mental health issues, the section on "Sexuality/Sex Therapy" provides useful general information on common problems and criteria for selecting a therapist.

Imerman Angels (www.imermanangels.org)—A source of free personalized connections that enable one-on-one support among cancer fighters, survivors, and caregivers; you are carefully matched with someone who has experienced your cancer and your issues, is the same gender, and is close in age to you.

New Health Advisor (www.newhealthadvisor.com)—Lively presentations in the Sex & Relationship section give answers to "Why do orgasms feel good?" and "How to get in the mood."

TED Talks (www.ted.com/talks)—Some of the best relationship and sex counselors in the world have shared their humor, inspiration, and expertise in these talks. The endnotes provide links to specific talks, but especially for our readers, we recommend those (in alphabetical order) by Brené Brown, Eve Ensler, Esther Perel, Mary Roach, and for the light touch, actress/comedienne Julia Sweeny.

Glossary

Alopecia—Partial or complete baldness; when induced by chemotherapy, it is rarely permanent.

Basal cell—A type of cell deep within the skin that produces new skin cells as old ones die. Basal cell carcinoma is a type of skin cancer with one, rare version of vulvar cancer falling into this category.

Brachytherapy—Internal radiation therapy.

Breast cancer—Presence of a tumor in the breast composed of cells that are able to invade surrounding tissues or spread to other areas of the body.

CA 125—Cancer antigen 125; a protein that may reach elevated levels in the blood of patients with certain types of cancers; most often associated with testing for ovarian cancer.

Carcinoma—A cancerous tumor that begins in the skin or in tissue covering an internal organ.

Cervical cancer—Cancer in the area of the body that connects the uterus to the vagina; nearly all cases are caused by human papillomavirus (HPV), therefore, they are preventable with the HPV vaccine.

Chemotherapy—Treatment using chemicals that have a toxic effect on the disease cells.

Cold cap—A cap worn during chemotherapy to prevent hair loss.

Conization—Using a surgical knife, laser knife, or a heated wire to remove a cone-shaped piece of tissue. Although this is often used as a diagnostic technique, it can also be used as a treatment for women with early stage cancer who want to preserve their ability to give birth.

Cryosurgery—The use of cold to kill abnormal cells.

Debulking surgery—Removal of as much of a tumor as possible.

Depressive realism—Hypothesis developed by psychologists Lauren Alloy and Lyn Yvonne Abramson that depressed individuals make more realistic inferences than do nondepressed individuals.

Dopamine—A chemical that functions as a neurotransmitter in the brain; high dopamine levels mean you are in tune with pleasure, whereas reduced dopamine levels mean that your perceptions of reward and pleasure are low.

Double voiding—A therapy to help people completely empty their bladders to avert a problem of leftover urine in the bladder that can cause pelvic pain and urine infections.

Ductal carcinoma in situ (DCIS)—The most common type of noninvasive breast cancer. The cancer starts inside the milk ducts. It's noninvasive because it hasn't spread beyond the milk ducts into the surrounding breast tissue, but the presence of it puts a woman at high risk for cancer coming back. With DCIS, the odds of a recurrence are about one in three.

Dyspareunia—Painful sexual intercourse.

Endometrial cancer—Cancer in the lining of the uterus; see also uterine cancer.

Endorphins—Hormones secreted within the brain and nervous system that activate opiate receptors; "feel good" hormones.

Epithelial—Describing a type of ovarian cancer in which the malignant cells are in the tissue covering the ovary.

Erotic intelligence—As defined by psychotherapist and sexuality expert Esther Perel (*Mating in Captivity: Unlocking Erotic Intelligence*), a state of being that has more to do with imagination than something primal and animalistic; it is rooted in curiosity, playfulness, and mystery.

External beam radiation therapy (EBRT)—Given like an X-ray, except that the radiation dose is significantly stronger.

Female sexual arousal disorder (FSAD)—Inability to achieve or maintain sexual excitement.

Female Sexual Function Index (FSFI)—A nineteen-question, multiple-choice test instrument that is a measure of sexual activity, sexual intercourse, and sexual stimulation.

Fistula—A permanent abnormal passageways between organs or between an organ and the exterior of the body.

G-spot—An erogenous area toward the top of the vagina; aka Gräfenberg spot.

Germ cells—Cells in the ovary, destined to form eggs, that are a potential source of malignancy.

Human papillomavirus (HPV)—Cause of cervical cancer as well as a few other cancers transmitted through intimate contact with an infected person; HPV vaccine is used to prevent it.

Hypertonic—In relation to sexual dysfunction, describing an abnormally high muscle tone that inhibits proper functioning of the pelvic floor muscles.

Hypoactive sexual desire disorder (HSDD)—A sexual dysfunction characterized by low sexual desire.

Hysterectomy—Removes the uterus and cervix; the three basic ways to do a hysterectomy are: (1) removal through the abdomen, (2) through the vagina, and (3) by using laparoscopy. A robotic assist is a common practice.

Immunotherapy—Treatment that employs substances that stimulate the body's own immune response.

Inorgasmia—Inability to experience orgasm.

Introitus—Entrance to the vagina.

Invasive cancer—The cancer cells have broken out of the small lobe where they began. They therefore have the potential to spread to the lymph nodes, which are part of the immune system.

Kegel exercises—Exercises to strengthen the pelvic floor muscles.

Laser surgery—A focused beam burns off abnormal cells or a piece of tissue; not used to treat invasive cancer.

Lobular carcinoma in situ (LCIS)—A marker for breast cancer, but not breast cancer; it is an area of abnormal cell growth that increases a person's risk of developing breast cancer later. "Lobular" means that the abnormal cells are in the lobules, or milk-producing glands.

Myofascial release—Hands-on treatment to help release tension of the fascia; that is, a thin covering of tissue enclosing a muscle or other organ.

Noninvasive cancer—The cancer cells are contained in the lobe where they began.

Omentum—A layer of fat that is covered by the peritoneum, the membrane lining the walls of the abdominal and pelvic cavities. The greater omentum attaches to the bottom part of the stomach and hangs in front of the intestines. The lesser omentum is attached to the top edge of the stomach and extends to the undersurface of the liver. In 80 percent of women, by the time ovarian cancer is diagnosed, it has spread to the omentum.

Ovarian cancer—Cancer in one or both of the glands that produce eggs for reproduction and the female hormones estrogen and progesterone.

Oxytocin—A hormone that appears to be released during orgasm as well as hugging, touching, pregnancy, childbirth, and breastfeeding; often referred to as the "love hormone" or "cuddle hormone," it is associated with a feeling of trust and connectedness, so it therefore reinforces a sense of comfort.

Pelvic exenteration—A radical surgery involving the removal of reproductive organs and tissues as well as others in the pelvic area.

Pelvic floor—Muscles at the base of the abdomen that support certain organs; their proper function is vital to urinary and fecal continence as well as sexual functioning.

Pelvic lymph node dissection—Surgery in response to a concern that cancer has spread from the original site; removal of lymph nodes while doing the hysterectomy or trachelectomy would either confirm or refute the suspicion.

Perineum—The area between the anus and the scrotum or vulva that is considered an erogenous zone.

Physiatry—A medical specialization in physical medicine and rehabilitation.

Positive illusion—A type of self-deception that helps people maintain a sense of well-being, even in the face of discomfort or threat.

Radiation oncology—Use of radiation in the treatment of cancer.

Sarcoma—A malignancy that begins in bone, cartilage, fat, muscle, blood vessels, or other connective tissue.

Sensate focus—The centerpiece of the clinical work done by Masters and Johnson; consists of exercises to increase awareness of one's own and a partner's intimacy needs.

Sexual response cycle—A phrase describing the three phases of a conventional sexual encounter: arousal, climax, and resolution.

Squamous cells—The primary type of skin cells.

Stages of cancer—The National Cancer Institute describes five stages: Stage 0 refers to carcinoma confined to its original site; Stages I, II, and III, respectively, indicate more extensive disease; Stage IV means the cancer has spread to distant tissues or organs.

Stromal cells—Hormone-releasing cells connecting the structures of the ovaries that can house malignancy.

Trachelectomy—Addresses certain Stage I cancers in a way that still allows the woman to have children.

Uterine cancer—Cancer in the lining of the uterus; see also endometrial cancer.

Vaginal brachytherapy—A source of radiation is placed into a cylinder and inserted into the vagina.

Vaginal cancer—Cancer of the three-to-four-inch muscular tube running from the cervix to the vulva.

Vaginal stenosis—The vagina becomes extremely narrow and inflexible.

Vulvar cancer—Cancer of the external part of the female genitalia; the fourth most common gynecologic cancer.

Notes

CHAPTER 1

1. "Cancer Staging: What Is Staging?" National Cancer Institute, National Institutes of Health, http://www.cancer.gov/about-cancer/diagnosis-staging/staging/staging-fact-sheet.

2. In 2013, the GAVI Alliance (formerly the Global Alliance for Vaccines and Immunisation) launched a demonstration program to provide HPV vaccines to 180,000 adolescent girls in eight countries. GAVI negotiated a cost for the vaccine that's less than $5 per dose, as opposed to the going rate at the time of $13 per dose. The group, with financial support for target countries from the Pan American Health Organization (PAHO) Revolving Fund, aims to make the vaccine available to thirty million girls in forty countries by 2020. See: http://deainfo.nci.nih.gov/advisory/pcp/annualReports/HPV/Part4.htm#sthash.T6aRvNuP.dpbs.

3. "Survival Rate for Cervical Cancer, by Stage," American Cancer Society, http://www.cancer.org/cancer/cervicalcancer/detailedguide/cervical-cancer-survival.

4. "Types and States of Ovarian Cancer," National Ovarian Cancer Coalition, http://www.ovarian.org/types_and_stages.php.

5. "What Are the Risk Factors for Ovarian Cancer?" http://www.cancer.org/cancer/ovariancancer/detailedguide/ovarian-cancer-risk-factors.

6. "What Is Vulvar Cancer?" American Cancer Society, http://www.cancer.org/cancer/vulvarcancer/detailedguide/vulvar-cancer-what-is-vulvar-cancer.

CHAPTER 2

1. I. E. Krop, M. Beeram, S. Modi, S. F. Jones, S. N. Holden, W. Yu, S. Girish, J. Tibbitts, J. H. Yi, M. X. Sliwkowski, F. Jacobson, S. G. Lutzker, and H. A. Burris, "Phase I Study of Trastuzumab-DM1, an HER2 Antibody-Drug Conjugate, Given

Every 3 Weeks to Patients with HER2-Positive Metastatic Breast Cancer," *Journal of Clinical Oncology* 28, no. 6 (June 2010): 2698–2704. (PMID: 20421541)

2. "What Are the Side Effects of Immunotherapy?" Dana-Farber Cancer Institute, March 8, 2016, http://blog.dana-farber.org/insight/2016/02/what-are-the-side-effects-of-immunotherapy/.

CHAPTER 3

1. P. A. Ganz, J. H. Rowland, K. Desmond, B. E. Meyerowitz, and G. E. Wyatt, "Life after Breast Cancer: Understanding Women's Health-Related Quality of Life and Sexual Functioning," *American Society of Clinical Oncology*, 1998, http://jco.ascopubs.org/content/16/2/501.short.

2. E. R. Greimel, R. Winter, K. S. Kapp, and J. Haas, "Quality of Life and Sexual Functioning after Cervical Cancer Treatment: A Long-Term Follow-Up Study," *Journal of Psychooncology* 18, no. 5 (2009): 476–82. doi: 10.1002/pon.1426; http://www.ncbi.nlm.nih.gov/pubmed/18702067.

3. Leslie R. Schover, Marleen van der Kaaij, Eleonora van Dorst, Carien Creutzberg, Eric Huyghe, and Cecilie E. Kiserud, "Sexual Dysfunction and Infertility as Late Effects of Cancer Treatment," *European Journal of Cancer Supplements* 12, no. 1 (June 2014): 41–53, 1st EORTC Cancer Survivorship Summit, http://www.sciencedirect.com/science/article/pii/S1359634914000068.

4. http://www.rand.org/health/surveys_tools/mos/36-item-short-form/survey-instrument.html.

5. http://cesd-r.com/.

6. Graham Spanier, PhD, "Dyadic Adjustment Scale," Multi-Health Services, http://www.mhs.com/product.aspx?gr=cli&prod=das&id=overview.

7. http://healthnet.umassmed.edu/mhealth/SexualFunction.pdf.

8. http://www.cancer.ucla.edu/patient-care/survivorship/for-healthcare-providers/cancer-rehabilitation-evaluation-system-cares.

9. "The Stigma of Hair Loss during Chemotherapy," uploaded by Sal Carty, September 10, 2015, https://www.youtube.com/watch?v=svaobs41Re4.

CHAPTER 4

1. "Know the Most Current Recommendations for PPE When Handling Hazardous Drugs," Oncology Nursing Society, https://www.ons.org/practice-resources/clinical-practice/know-most-current-recommendations-ppe-when-handling-hazardous.

2. "DCIS—Ductal Carcinoma In Situ," BreastCancer.org, http://www.breastcancer.org/symptoms/types/dcis.

3. Robert M. Sapolsky, "How to Relieve Stress," March 22, 2012, http://greatergood.berkeley.edu/article/item/how_to_relieve_stress.

4. Ibid.

5. Robert Sapolsky, PhD, as interviewed in the broadcast "Stress," Radiolab, NPR, Season 1, Episode 2, http://www.radiolab.org/story/91580-stress/.

6. Ibid.

CHAPTER 5

1. Melissa Conrad Stoppler, MD, Medical Editor: William C. Shiel Jr., MD, FACP, FACR, "CA 125," MedicineNet.com, http://www.medicinenet.com/ca_125/article.htm.

2. "FDA Approval for Gemcitabine Hydrochloride," National Cancer Institute, http://www.cancer.gov/about-cancer/treatment/drugs/fda-gemcitabine hydrochloride.

CHAPTER 6

1. Jeanette Scott, "Inorgasmia: Female Sexual Problem," *Consumer Health Digest*, https://www.consumerhealthdigest.com/female-sexual-health/inorgasmia.html.

2. Andrew Solomon, "Depression, the Secret We Share," TEDxMet, October 2013, https://www.ted.com/talks/andrew_solomon_depression_the_secret_we_share/transcript?language=en.

3. Shelley Taylor, "Adjustment to Threatening Events: A Theory of Cognitive Adaptation," *American Psychologist* 38, no. 11 (1983): 1161–73. doi:10.1037/0003-066X.38.11.1161

4. Shelley E. Taylor and David A. Armor, "Positive Illusions and Coping with Adversity," *Journal of Personality* 64, no. 4 (December 1996): 893 [pp. 873–98].

CHAPTER 7

1. From an interview with Trevor Crow Mullineaux, August 30, 2016.

2. Daniel J. Siegel, "Emotion as Integration: A Possible Answer to the Question, What Is Emotion?" in *The Healing Power of Emotion: Affective Neuroscience, Development & Clinical Practice*, eds. Diana Fosha, Daniel J. Siegel, Marion F. Solomon (New York: W. W. Norton, 2009), 148–49.

3. Michelle Wheeler quoting Matt Tilley, "Why Science Says You Should Have More Sex," MedicalXpress, August 29, 2016, http://medicalxpress.com/news/2016-08-science-sex.html.

4. Ibid.

5. Mullineaux interview, ibid.

6. "Sensate Focus Exercise: Non-Sexual Intimacy," http://www3.nd.edu/~pmtrc/Handouts/Sensate_Focus.pdf.

7. Yvonne K. Fulbright, PhD, "FOXSexpert: Touch Me There—The Rules of Sensate Focus Sex," Fox News, April 27, 2009, http://www.foxnews.com/story/2009/04/27/foxexpert-touch-me-there-rules-sensate-focus-sex.html.

8. Brené Brown, "The Power of Vulnerability," TEDxHouston, June 2010, https://www.ted.com/talks/brene_brown_on_vulnerability#t-444247.

9. Interview with Lynne Cox by Robin Young on *Here and Now*, WBUR, National Public Radio, August 31, 2016, http://www.wbur.org/hereandnow/2016/08/31/lynne-cox.

10. Ibid.

11. Brown, ibid.

12. Laura Trice, "Remember to Say Thank You," TED2008, February 2008, https://www.ted.com/talks/laura_trice_suggests_we_all_say_thank_you/transcript?language=en.

13. Esther Perel, "The Secret to Desire in a Long-Term Relationship," TEDSalon NY2013, February 2013, https://www.ted.com/talks/esther_perel_the_secret_to_desire_in_a_long_term_relationship/transcript?language=en.

14. Ruth Westheimer, EdD, interviewed by Lisa Zamosky in "Sex: Why Foreplay Matters (Especially for Women)," WebMD Magazine, http://www.webmd.com/sex-relationships/features/sex-why-foreplay-matters-especially-for-women.

15. It should also be noted that, in a 2013 experiment replicating the protocols, Coan found that women in what we would call a "bad marriage" were not calmed by holding their husband's hand; in fact, they felt more threatened.

16. James A. Coan, "Toward a Neuroscience of Attachment," in *Handbook of Attachment: Theory, Research, and Clinical Implications* (2nd Edition), eds. Jude Cassidy and Philip R. Shaver (New York: The Guildford Press, 2010), 260.

17. Trevor Crow (Mullineaux) and Maryann Karinch, *Forging Healthy Connections: How Relationships Fight Illness, Aging and Depression* (Far Hills, NJ: New Horizon Press, 2013), 126.

18. Perel, ibid.

19. Interview with Julia Bunning, DPT, on September 2, 2016.

20. Richard C. Bump, MD, W. Glenn Hurt, MD, J. Andrew Fantl, MD, and Jean F. Wyman, PhD, "Assessment of Kegel Pelvic Muscle Exercise Performance after Brief Verbal Instruction," *American Journal of Obstetrics & Gynecology* 165, no. 2 (August 1991): 322–29.

21. "Pelvic Floor Muscle (Kegel) Exercises for Women to Improve Sexual Health," Memorial Sloan Kettering Cancer Center, https://www.mskcc.org/cancer-care/patient-education/pelvic-floor-muscle-kegel-exercises-women-improve-sexual-health.

22. Interview with Lisa M. Ruppert, MD, on September 9, 2016.

23. "Double Voiding Technique," Kegel8, http://www.kegel8.co.uk/glossary/term/double-voiding-technique/.

24. http://www.pudendalhope.info/node/11.

25. Ibid.

26. Gert Holstege, MD, PhD, as quoted by Madeline Haller in "The 5 Craziest Sex Studies Ever," *Women's Health*, October 1, 2012, http://www.womenshealthmag.com/sex-and-love/the-5-craziest-sex-studies-ever.

27. "Attention Singles: Brooks Running Survey Reveals Majority Believe Running Increases Sex Appeal," BrooksRunning.com, June 4, 2012, https://www.brooksrunning.com/en_us/06-04-2014.html.

CHAPTER 8

1. International Couples Study on Satisfaction and Happiness, *Kinsey Today* (Late Summer 2011), https://kinseyinstitute.org/news-events/newsletters/pdf/Summer_2011_newsletter.pdf.

2. Holly N. Thomas, MD, Chung-Chou H. Chang, PhD, Stacey Dillon, MS, and Rachel Hess, MD, MS, "Sexual Activity in Midlife Women: Importance of Sex Matters," *JAMA Internal Medicine* 174, no. 4 (2014): 631–33. doi:10.1001/jamainternmed.2013.14402; https://archinte.jamanetwork.com/article.aspx?articleid=1828742.

3. Ibid.

4. Ruppert interview, ibid.

5. Interview with Jennifer A. Skyler, PhD, September 14, 2016.

6. Ibid.

7. Amy Gamerman, "One Writer Takes the New Female Viagra for a Spin," *Vogue*, December 18, 2015, http://www.vogue.com/13374393/female-viagra-addyi-results/.

8. Ibid.

9. "Antidepressant Use in Persons Aged 12 and Over: United States, 2005–2008," NCHS Data Brief No. 76, October 2011, Centers for Disease Control and Prevention, http://www.cdc.gov/nchs/data/databriefs/db76.htm.

10. Alessandro Serretti, MD, PhD, and Alberto Chiesa, MD, "Treatment-Emergent Sexual Dysfunction Related to Antidepressants: A Meta-Analysis," *Journal of Clinical Psychopharmocology* 29, no. 3 (June 2009), http://www.medapharma.cz/pdf/Aurorix-1-2009-SD-metaanalysis-Serretti-A-Chiesays.pdf.

11. Daniel J. DeNoon, "Viagra Improves Sex for Some Women," WebMD, referencing J. R. Berman in *The Journal of Urology* 170 (December 2003): 2333–38, http://www.webmd.com/sexual-conditions/news/20040107/viagra-improves-sex-for-some-women#1.

12. Rabbi Shmuley Boteach, "Sex Tips from a Rabbi," YouTube, published October 2, 2012, https://www.youtube.com/watch?v=xrhYLjoQXGo.

13. Ibid.

14. Ruppert interview, ibid.

CONCLUSION

1. Eve Ensler, "Suddenly, My Body," TEDWomen 2010, December 2010, https://www.ted.com/talks/eve_ensler?language=en.

APPENDIX A

1. Interview with Jeanene Smith, associate director of the Colorado Ovarian Cancer Alliance, September 21, 2016.

Index

About the Authors

Saketh Guntupalli, MD, FACS, FACOG, is Vice Chairman for Clinical Affairs and Quality in the Department of Obstetrics and Gynecology at the University of Colorado School of Medicine at Denver. He is the principal investigator for the Gynecologic Oncology Group (GOG)/NRG research consortium for the University of Colorado and also serves as the director of the fellowship program in gynecologic oncology. Board certified in gynecologic oncology and obstetrics/gynecology, he is the recipient of two large grants to examine sexual dysfunction in women with cancer as well as post-operative quality outcomes. Guntupalli also serves as director for the Placenta Accreta Response Team (PART) at the University of Colorado Hospital. He has a focused interest in minimally invasive surgery, such as robotics and laparoscopy, as well as novel, molecular therapeutics in the treatment of gynecologic cancer. He has authored over forty clinical papers in journals such as the *Journal of the National Cancer Institute*, *Obstetrics and Gynecology*, *Gynecologic Oncology*, and the *International Journal of Gynecologic Oncology*.

Maryann Karinch is the author of twenty-six books, most of which focus on human health and behavior. In recognition of her work as a dedicated explorer of the psyche and mind-body interaction, The Explorers Club took an unusual step and elected her to membership in 2010. She is also a member of The Authors Guild. In 2004, Karinch founded The Rudy Agency, a literary agency, representing the full range of fiction and nonfiction. Among the international media outlets that have covered Karinch's human behavior work are ABC News, *Boston Globe*, *Christian Science Monitor*, *Fast Company*, Huffington Post, *Washington Post*, *New York Daily News*, and NPR.